DATE DUE

GAYLORD			PRINTED IN U.S.A.

ISLAMIC SURVEYS 11

ISLAMIC MEDICINE

Manfred Ullmann

at the
EDINBURGH
University Press

EDINBURGH
UNIVERSITY
PRESS
22
George Square
Edinburgh
ISBN
0 85224 325 1
Printed in
Great Britain
by R. & R. Clark, Ltd.,
Edinburgh

FOREWORD

This series of Islamic Surveys was launched about fourteen years ago with the aim of 'giving the educated reader something more than can be found in the usual popular books'. The general idea was that each work should survey some part of the vast field covered by Islamic Studies, not merely presenting an outline of what was known and generally accepted, but also indicating the points at which scholarly debate continued. A bibliography, preferably annotated, was to guide the reader who wished to pursue his study further. The series has advanced more slowly than was hoped, but to judge from the reception of the volumes so far published, the general aim has been realized fairly well. We have not yet managed to include in the series all the volumes we should have liked to include, and we have added some that were not originally thought of.

We are specially pleased to add this eleventh volume to the series, since there is no recent book on the subject in any European language. The state of scholarship at present places certain limitations on the treatment, as the author explains; and in this we must follow his judgement, since he, more than anyone else, is familiar with the source material in all its variety and vast extent. Despite the limitations, however, this book is an important contribution to Islamic studies, and its authoritative character will commend it also to those interested in the history of medicine.

As in other volumes of the series, the transliteration of Arabic words is essentially that of the second edition of *The Encyclopaedia of Islam* (London, 1960, continuing) with three modifications. Two of these are normal with most British Arabists, namely, *q* for *ḳ*, and *j* for *dj*. The third is something of a novelty. It is the replacement of the ligature used to show when two consonants are to be sounded together by an apostrophe to show when they are to be sounded separately. This means that *dh*, *gh*, *kh*, *sh*, *th* are to be sounded together; where there is an apostrophe, as in *ad'ham*, they are to be sounded separately. The apostrophe in this usage represents no sound, but, since it only occurs between two consonants (of which the second is *h*), it cannot be confused with the apostrophe representing the glottal stop (*hamza*), which never occurs between two consonants.

W. Montgomery Watt

THE CONTENTS

THE ILLUSTRATIONS

The publisher is grateful to the various libraries and institutions for permission to reproduce the illustrations.

INTRODUCTION

The book that I here give to the public bears the title *Islamic Medicine.* It is the account of a medical system which was introduced into Arab countries in the ninth century A.D. and was practised throughout the Middle Ages and right up to modern times. This system is widely known under the term 'Arabian Medicine'. But many doctors, among them some of the most outstanding like ar-Rāzī (Rhazes), al-Majūsī (Haly Abbas) and Ibn-Sīnā (Avicenna), were Persians, not Arabs. To be sure, they wrote their scientific works chiefly in Arabic. On the other hand, there were many doctors who were Christians, like Ḥunayn ibn-Is'ḥāq, or Jews, like Maimonides. But their religious allegiance is in this context just as irrelevant as their ethnic origins. All these scholars lived within the sphere of Islamic culture and have helped in a most enduring way to shape this culture and to give it its particular stamp. So when we talk of 'Islamic Medicine', we are thinking of Islam as a cultural force; we are looking at a culture which has absorbed many different currents within itself and integrated and developed them.

'Islamic medicine' did not grow on Arab soil. Rather it is the medicine of later Greek antiquity which was formulated in the Arabic language in the South and West of the Mediterranean from the ninth century A.D. The crossing of the language barrier has left the contents almost completely unchanged. Medicine, along with philosophy, mathematics, astronomy and astrology, not to mention zoology and alchemy, geography and technology, belongs to those disciplines which have Hellenized the Arab-Islamic world. The hellenization which then took place was one of the great universal historical movements, whose effects are felt to this day. Francesco Gabrieli has rightly said that 'the struggle for the incorporation into Islam... of the thought of antiquity belongs to the most exciting chapters of its intellectual history'.[1] Attempts have been made in many works to interpret this process of Hellenization but in detail much is still very obscure. Too many real facts are still unknown; the greater part of the problem is until now unexplored.

In the field of medicine, the manuscript tradition has preserved for us a vast number of sources but by far the largest part of these sources has not yet been edited. Those works that have been published present almost without exception uncritical and inaccurate texts. Therefore 'the student of Arabic medical literature must' as Edward Granville Browne said 55 years ago 'begin by correcting and re-editing even the printed texts before he can begin to read or translate them'.[2] These conditions make it almost impossible, even to-day, to write the history of Islamic medicine. The literature that is available is therefore seen to be scanty enough even when considered in its entirety.

Even to-day we must return to the two-volume work *Histoire de la médecine arabe* by Lucien Leclerc (Paris, 1876; reprinted New York, n.d., ? 1960). Leclerc aimed at writing the complete history of Arabic medicine so as to show its origins, its character, its institutions, its development and its decay. He realized, however, that he could only provide an 'external' or 'bio-bibliographic' history. He relied extensively on the Arabic book catalogues and biographical works, that is, on the *Fihrist* of Ibn-an-Nadīm, the *Ta'rīkh al-ḥukamā'* of al-Qifṭī and on the *'Uyūn* of Ibn-Abī-Uṣaybi'a, whose contents he reproduced in long dry lists. Still valuable to-day are those parts of his book in which he describes the results of his studies of manuscripts undertaken at the Bibliothèque Nationale in Paris and in the Escorial.

A valuable and, for that period, very noteworthy little book is *Arabian Medicine* by the above-mentioned E. G. Browne.[3] Browne made a few major works the object of his researches: the *Paradise of Wisdom* of 'Alī ibn-Sahl aṭ-Ṭabarī, the *Kitāb al-Ḥāwī* of ar-Rāzī (*Continens* of Rhazes), the *Kitāb al-Malakī* (*Liber Regius*) of 'Alī ibn-al-'Abbās al-Majūsī, the *Qānūn* of Ibn-Sīnā (*Canon* of Avicenna) and the *Dhakhīra* of Ismā'īl al-

Jurjānī written in Persian. In the opening chapter in which Browne describes the beginnings of medicine among the Arabs, he has accepted assertions of the Arabic tradition which have not stood up to historical criticism.

The English reader has also available the book by Cyril Elgood, *A Medical History of Persia and the Eastern Caliphate from the Earliest Times until the Year* A.D. *1932* (Cambridge 1951). This is a comprehensive work dealing both with Persian medicine and the classical period of Arabic or Islamic medicine. The book suffers a little from a lack of historical method and is not always reliable in details but the very exact information about the development of Persian medicine in the last centuries is extremely valuable.

In the years 1970 and 1971 there appeared two books which attempted to assess Arabic medical literature as far as this exists in manuscripts or fragments. One is *Die Medizin im Islam* by the present writer,[4] the other is the third volume of the *Geschichte des arabischen Schrifttums* by Fuat Sezgin.[5] Whereas the presentation in the first book continues into the seventeenth century, Sezgin deals only with the period up to A.D. 1040. Sezgin's material is in part more comprehensive than the present author's, but the evaluation of this material and its historical arrangement would seem to be problematic.[6] Both books, *Medizin im Islam* and *GAS*, are essentially bibliographical works of reference which should provide the foundations for further research. They do not contain a history of medical theory.

This present small book is in line with the state of contemporary research by avoiding the word 'history' in its title. Its terms of reference are limited. This means that important areas like surgery and hospital institutions, and questions like the doctor's social standing, the doctor-patient relationship, or medical teaching, will not be discussed; and from the multitude of interesting medical theories, only a few can be selected and presented. However, it seemed right to me to deal with a few specially characteristic subjects in fuller detail and to give prominence to anything of outstanding significance. So I have described the Hellenization process in considerable detail, I have stressed Islamic medicine's dependence on tradition and have spent some time on the problem of the relation of rational medicine to magic and astrology. I have also described what the medieval doctor knew about human physiology. The dry schematism of that physiological system may perhaps put off the modern reader. But he must be acquainted with this system if he is to be able to understand Arabic medical literature. 'Islamic medicine' is the discipline of a period which knew no Renaissance and no Enlightenment. One must therefore be careful not to measure it with the same yardstick that one would apply to the history of European disciplines.

This present volume is written by a philologist who is neither a doctor nor a medical historian. For this reason doctors may feel that he has not tackled many questions which seem to them important. However, the author hopes that where he had to deal with medical subjects beyond the sphere of philology or history, he will not be considered to have fallen too far short of the mark.

This book has been written at the suggestion of Professor Montgomery Watt, the editor of the series. My warmest thanks to him for all his trouble. My warmest thanks also to his wife, Dr Jean Watt, who has made an excellent translation of the book into English. And, finally, I would like to express to the staff of Edinburgh University Press my deep gratitude for their careful and accurate work.

evil eye (*al-ʿayn*) was considered a reality. Magic spells were for the most part prohibited; they were, however, allowed if someone had been affected by the evil eye or had been stung by a snake or scorpion. Expectoration, on the other hand, might help in a case of bewitchment.[21]

None of this is very important. It is the usual folk-medicine which is found in all primitive societies *mutatis mutandis*. However, these ideas have acquired a great significance in later Islamic history. Because they were held to be the teachings of the Prophet, they were collected and combined with many late unauthentic Ḥadīth and then interpreted by using the concepts of Greek medicine. The end product of all these methods was called 'Prophetic Medicine' (*aṭ-ṭibb an-nabawī*) and was to counter Hellenistic Greek medicine which for orthodoxy was suspect as being a science of heathen origin. This prophetic medicine certainly met with strong response from the people. Ibn-Khaldūn alone has said clearly that essentially this is bedouin medicine and can have no claim to be divine revelation and therefore cannot be obligatory under religious law.[22]

If one leaves out the Ḥadīth, there is very little known about medicine in the early Islamic and the Umayyad periods (661–750). Something can be learnt from anecdotes. ʿUrwa ibn-az-Zubayr ibn-al-ʿAwwām, for example, in the year 704 while staying in Syria with the later caliph al-Walīd ibn-ʿAbd-al-Malik, is said to have contracted gangrene of the foot (*ikla*). His foot was amputated in al-Walīd's presence but ʿUrwa uttered no cry so that al-Walīd only knew that the operation was over when he smelt the burning of the cauterization with which the wound was treated afterwards. ʿUrwa lived for another eight years. This is recorded by Ibn-Qutayba.[23] In the parallel account of Abū-l-Faraj al-Iṣfahānī[24] it is also told how they wanted to give ʿUrwa a pain-killer, but ʿUrwa refused this as being beneath his dignity. However, this is probably only a legendary embellishing of the account.

Wahb ibn-Munabbih, about whose life nothing reliable is known (he is said to have died about 732),[25] had perhaps certain ideas about human physiology as taught by the Greeks. He speaks of the four primary qualities and the four humours related to them and of the balance of temperament which signifies health. He located the mental powers in particular organs:

intellect in the brain, greed in the kidneys, anger in the liver, courage in the heart, fear in the lungs, laughter in the spleen, sadness and joy in the face. Man was thought to have 360 members. He claimed to have found all this information in the Old Testament where they were said to be quoted in connection with the creation of Adam.[26]

The poet al-Farazdaq (d. 728) uses the word *mā'*, 'water' to denote an eye complaint.[27] Here too, Greek influence may be present because the words *hypokhyma* or *katarraktēs* 'cataract' were later represented in translation literature as *nuzūl al-mā'*, 'the descent of the water', or simply *al-mā'*.

Three doctors are said to have lived at that time who presumably practised a type of Hellenistic medicine. One of them, Tiyādhūq, is said to have been physician to the governor al-Ḥajjāj ibn-Yūsuf;[28] the other, Māsarjawayh, is said to have been of Persian-Jewish descent and to have lived in Basra. The third, Isrā'īl, was physician to the caliph Sulaymān ibn-'Abd-al-Malik (715–17). But the reports about these men are very unclear and full of contradictions so that one cannot take anything from them with certainty. It is quite clear, however, that the scientific doctors at that time were Greeks, Persians, Syrians, or Jews. But in addition there always existed folk-medicine. The grammarian Yūnus ibn-Ḥabīb (d. 798) used to avail himself frequently of aloes because he believed they smoothed the skin, cleared away pimples, and purified the nerves.[29]

TWO

THE AGE OF THE TRANSLATIONS

After the death of the prophet Muḥammad in 632 and the defeat of the tribes of central Arabia which had revolted against Islam, we come to the unparalleled expansion of the Arabs: within a century they had created an empire from Spain to the valley of the Indus. With Egypt, Syria, Mesopotamia and Persia, countries had fallen to them whose population had reached a high level of culture, which was shot through with Hellenism and thus in certain areas presented a relatively uniform picture.

After the Near East had been more and more christianized, Koine-Greek lost in significance in this area as lingua franca, while the native languages, Aramaic in Syria and Iraq, Coptic in Egypt, and Pahlavi in Persia, flourished again. Since intellectuals and scholars no longer always understood Greek, the need became apparent to translate the Greek works into the national languages. The christianization of the colleges in the sixth century also resulted in a shift of syllabus. Whereas previously Greek poetry, tragedy and historiography were taught and explained, as well as philosophy, medicine and the exact sciences, the syllabus was now reduced to the latter subjects because only these were relevant for the new religious beliefs and useful for the life-style. Thus when the Arabs later became the 'secondary-modern pupils' of the Greeks, this was not because they were not interested in humanistic subjects but because the stream of these subjects had already dried up. The Arabs could only acquire that part of the Greek corpus of learning which the Christians in Syria and Egypt were then in a position to offer.

The late period of the University of Alexandria from the fourth to the seventh centuries shows up these tendencies in detail. Aristotelian exegesis had produced outstanding figures in Ammonius, John Philoponus, David, Elias and Stephanus. Less is known about the medical teachers. Palladius and Asclepius explained some writings of Hippocrates in the sixth century. However, after the conquest of Alexandria by the Arabs in 642, the school remained in existence until about 719. Even under Muslim rule the Greek language was probably still in use for teaching and writing. This would explain why we have only the Arabic translations of the synopsis of the sixteen basic works of Galen, or of the book on pediatrics by Paul of Aegina. Greek manuscripts of these works could obviously no longer reach Constantinople because the political boundaries were now different. This is why Gessius, Anqīlāwus, John and Marinus, the editors of Galen's writings, cannot be more closely identified. Their names are only known from Arabic sources. It is quite uncertain whether these doctors were joined by Arabs as is related of ʿAbd-al-Malik ibn-Abjar al-Kinānī, who is said to have become personal physician to the caliph ʿUmar ibn-ʿAbd-al-ʿAzīz (*regnabat* 717–20).

The Umayyad caliphs retained the system of administration and other institutions in the conquered countries, that is to say, they simply took them over, but they could not concern themselves with the appropriation of Hellenistic culture because their attention was taken up externally by the conquests, and internally with strengthening the empire. This state of affairs completely changed after the take-over by the Abbasid caliphs and the founding of Baghdad. The Hellenization of Islam which now began received a strong impulse from Islamic theology, since the theologians made use of the weapon of Greek dialectic and logic in order to give the Islamic religion a dogmatic basis. Builders and engineers used Greek mathematics and mechanics, and the geographers the *Geōgraphikē Hyphēgēsis* of Ptolemy; and similarly for practical reasons interest was aroused in astronomy, astrology and alchemy. Medicine, too, belongs in this context.

Greek works

Before the year 800, translations were few and scanty but after that Greek works were received in an undreamt-of degree.

logical thinking that seeks to recognize and explain each organ and each natural process in terms of its purpose. Finally, to Galen can be traced back that rationalism that has left its impress on most Arabic writings.

The tradition of Hippocrates only followed in the shadow of Galen. The name of Hippocrates was indeed also famous among the Arabs and when ʿAbd-ar-Raḥmān ibn-ʿAlī ibn-Abī-Ṣādiq from Nīshāpūr (d. after 1068) was called the 'second Hippocrates' this was a title of great honour which he shares with Diocles of Carystus. The fact that the Hippocratic oath was demanded from the Arab doctors shows how strongly and for how long medical ethics were tied to his name. It was indeed known that several authors were involved in the *Corpus hippocraticum*. Thābit ibn-Qurra believed there were four authors called Hippocrates whose writings were combined in the editing. He calls them the Buqrāṭiyyūn, just as we talk of 'Hippocratics'.[4] But the interest of the translators and their patrons in Hippocrates was far less than in Galen. Important works like the great gynaecological writings *De morbis muliebribus*, *De natura muliebri*, *De sterilibus* and *De septimestri partu* remained untranslated, and when a minor work like *De superfetatione* was translated into Arabic,[5] it was almost by chance. There are indeed Arabic manuscripts of the *Aphorisms* and of the writings *De natura hominis*, *De officina medici* and *De aere aquis locis*, but in the case of these texts it is not a question of independently prepared translations but of the lemmata of Galen's commentaries which were excerpted and then transmitted in secondary fashion. This process of secondary transmission of the lemmata was repeated in the case of Palladius, an Alexandrian Iatrosophist of the sixth century. His commentary on the *Aphorisms* was translated, and when the historian al-Yaʿqūbī (*c.* 872) handed on sixty-three aphorisms of Hippocrates, he selected them from this commentary only.[6] Simply for this reason relatively unimportant Alexandrian commentators were of greater importance for the Arabs than Hippocrates himself, because they were nearer in time and because they presented more simply the contents of the difficult Hippocratic writings dressed up in the spirit of Galen. There was no dearth of manuscripts of these commentaries whereas original Hippocratica had become in part quite scarce. So it need not surprise us that the large two-volume work *De morbis muliebribus* was not translated into Arabic, and that on the other hand, the Arabs possessed in translation two commentaries to the *De muliebribus* from the late Alexandrian period: the one was wrongly ascribed to Galen, the other originated in a doctor named Asclepius who was a pupil of the neoplatonic philosopher Ammonius, son of Hermeias.

The case of the Hippocratic writing *De victu* which was not translated in its entirety is also characteristic. The quotations from it which we find in a number of Arab authors, go back, as Dr Rainer Degen has shown, to the *Kitāb al-Aghdhiya* of Ḥunayn ibn-Is'ḥāq, in the drafting of which Ḥunayn had specially adapted or translated passages from *De victu* which served his purpose. In general the basic elements of his *Kitāb al-Aghdhiya* are taken from Galen's book *De alimentorum facultatibus*.

Mutatis mutandis, what had already taken place in the time of the Roman Empire and was to occur again in medieval Europe, repeated itself in the Islamic world of the ninth century, namely, the fact that the transmission of Hippocratic medicine was decisively furthered by Galen's works, and that Hippocrates owed the prestige he enjoyed largely to Galen.

Arabic pharmacology received its strongest impulse through the *Materia medica* of Dioscurides (written *c.* A.D. 77) of which not only the five original books but also the apocryphal books VI and VII on poisonous plants and animals were translated. The most widely circulated was the version prepared by Iṣṭafān ibn-Bāsīl and revised by Ḥunayn ibn-Is'ḥāq. Even today it is preserved in numerous manuscripts, often very beautifully illuminated;[7] it was used by nearly all Arab doctors and pharmacologists, indeed in part quoted from so extensively that it must be reckoned among the best-transmitted Arabic books. Al-Bīrūnī (d. 1048), who, when over 80, joined with Aḥmad ibn-Muhammad an-Nahshaʿī to write an important pharmaceutical work,[8] praises the outstanding zeal for research of this Greek: 'If Dioscurides had lived in our country and had turned his efforts into determining the effects of the plants in our hills and valleys, these would have been used as medicines (*adwiya*) and the fruits would, as the result of his experiences, have become medicaments (*ashfiya*)'.

Also significant was the influence of Rufus of Ephesus, a doctor in Trajan's time, of whose writings no fewer than fifty-eight have been translated into Arabic. In them he dealt with many pathological and dietetic questions, discussed kidney and bladder disease, arthritis, jaundice, melancholy, hygiene of children, of young girls and of travellers, the art of anamnesis, the naming of the parts of the human body and much else besides.

In the same way, Philagrius, who lived in the fourth century A.D. produced many monographs in which he discussed especially the problems of internal illnesses. More than a dozen of these writings have been translated into Arabic, as also writings on consumption, sciatica, gout, stomach pains, cholic, diabetes, dropsy and attacks of hysterical choking.

Crito had worked as Trajan's personal physician in Rome at the turn of the first to the second century. His main work, the *Kosmētika*, which, as was then the custom, dealt with the whole range of skin diseases, was translated. The translation, however, has been lost in its entirety as has also the original Greek. The numerous Arabic fragments which have been preserved for us by ar-Rāzī, al-Baladī, Ibn-al-Jazzār and other doctors, supplement for us in the happiest fashion the passages that Galen incorporated into his work *De compositione medicamentorum*.

It was probably in the second century A.D. that Antyllus lived, who gained great recognition for himself especially in the field of surgery.[9] His *Kheirurgumena* were also translated into Arabic as well as a small surgical writing of Plato, a doctor of the pre-Galenic period, who had specialized in the use of the cauterizing iron.

Also a whole series of treatises on uroscopy, a much-practised and greatly overrated diagnostic method, have been translated. We know four authors by name, namely, Magnus, Pythagoras, Stephanus and Archelaus, who probably lived in the sixth century A.D.

Finally, we must mention the four great Byzantine compilators: Oribasius (326–403), personal physician to Julian the Apostate, Aetius of Amida who was active at the time of Justinian (*regnabat* 527–67), Alexander of Tralles (d. 605) and Paul of Aegina who lived at the time of Heraclius I (*regnabat*

610–41) and probably experienced personally how Alexandria fell into the hands of the Arabs in 642. Their works have had an influence on Arabic medicine which cannot yet be assessed. Their literary form, the great all-embracing total presentation of medicine, was imitated by ar-Rāzī, Aḥmad ibn-Muḥammad aṭ-Ṭabarī, al-Majūsī, Ibn-Sīnā, az-Zahrāwī, Ibn-Hubal and by many others. Surgery and midwifery were treated in depth after the model of the sixth book of Paul of Aegina.[10] In pathological questions, Galen's work *De locis affectis* did not always serve as a source but often the work of Aetius in which Galen's teachings merged with those of other doctors. The great compendia worked in the same way as the *Summaria Alexandrinorum*, that is to say, they presented the material in a form which went beyond Galen and was more comprehensive but partly also too diluted. The *Collectiones medicae* of Oribasius were never very widely circulated among the Arabs because of their enormous bulk. They too were chiefly influenced by Galen;[11] they also familiarized the Arabs with extracts from many other Greek authors belonging to other schools of thought like Erasistratus, Herophilus, Diocles of Carystus, Athenaeus, Mnesitheus, Dieuches, etc. To what extent the Arab doctors consciously absorbed into their system those deviant schools of thought, will be explained later. Finally, the great therapeutic work of Alexander of Tralles allowed the Arabs a glimpse into Hellenistic magic which is more strongly emphasized by this author than by the others.[12]

Alexander's work, however, was not the only book to acquaint the Arabs with magic. In addition, a whole number of hermetic writings has been translated, for example the *Kyranis*, which shows how to make amulets from a stone, a bird, a fish and a plant, and these can then be used to perform magic rites and cures.[13] The magical and healing effects of the stones have been described in a book by Xenocrates of Ephesus (first century A.D.), translated into Arabic at the beginning of the ninth century and prototype for many other similar writings, to which the famous pseudo-Aristotelian book of stones belongs.[14] In the last chapter of this book we shall deal with the question of how the Arab doctors were able to combine the rationalist medicine of Galen with occultism.

When one reads all that the Arabs had translated from the

Greek, one is rightly impressed by the wealth of medical knowledge which at that time was transplanted into another world. Many hundreds of works were arabized in the course of the ninth century giving one at first the impression that the Arabs took over the Greek medicine in its totality. But it must not be forgotten that there was a limit to these attempts, and it must be remembered that certain Greek authors did not reach the Arabs. It has already been noted that a whole number of the works of Hippocrates remained completely unknown and that others were only translated by the circuitous means of Galen's commentaries, that Hippocrates, so to speak, only came to the Arabs trailing behind Galen. The great Alexandrian anatomists of the third century B.C., Erasistratus and Herophilus, were at the time of Ḥunayn no longer obtainable in manuscript, so the Arabs were only indirectly acquainted with these doctors through Galen's criticisms and the excerpts of Oribasius.[15] The work too, of Aretaeus of Cappadocia, *De causis et signis morborum acutorum et chronicorum* was not translated because already in later antiquity it was used and quoted only by few doctors; the reason for this may have been the archaizing Ionic in which he wrote.[16] Unfortunately as a result the Arabs did not get to know the excellent, lively, exact and fascinating descriptions of illnesses and their symptoms provided by Aretaeus. It was perhaps only by chance that Soranus was not translated. Soranus, who lived in Ephesus at the beginning of the second century, was the most significant representative of the 'methodical' school and his work was the most important gynaecological writing of antiquity. In the Western medieval world, Soranus always ranked third after Galen and Hippocrates; in the East, on the other hand, only the most meagre bits of information were associated with his name.

Syriac works

The fact that within a century Greek medicine became so strongly indigenous among the Arabs, can be partly explained by the fact that it was received into a soil that had already been Hellenized for centuries.

The translation of Greek medical works into Syriac was accomplished chiefly in two periods. The best-known figure of the earlier epoch was Sergius of Rēsh-ʿAynā (d. 536) who had translated numerous writings by Galen. The second epoch came three hundred years later. It is distinguished by names like Job of Edessa (d. after 832) and Ḥunayn and his pupils. It therefore already coincides with the great cultural movement among the Abbasid caliphs and it must not be forgotten that at that time many Greek works were translated into Arabic from Syriac and not directly from the Greek.

But the Syrians did not confine themselves purely to the role of mediator. Being conversant with the concepts and content of Greek medicine, they had published independent writings in their own language which were then translated in the ninth century into Arabic in the same way as were the Syriac versions of Greek works. Among these were a book on dropsy by Sergius of Rēsh-ʿAynā, a book on uroscopy by Job of Edessa, and three compendia of general medicine, whose publishers were Shlēmōn, Shemʿōn d-Ṭaybūtheh and Yōḥannān bar Serāphyōn (John, son of Serapion).[17] The latter's work was translated three times into Arabic and later from Arabic into Latin where it often appeared, and was widely circulated, under the title *Practica Joannis Serapionis aliter breviarium nuncupata*.

Persian works

The lines of transmission that led from Greece through the Persian empire to the Arabs were similar to those in the Syrian world. In the Achaemenian empire, Greek doctors as well as Egyptian doctors had been prized at the court and had been preferred to the Persian practitioners of a magical and religious medicine. The best-known of these Greeks were Democedes of Croton whom Darius I (*regnabat* 521–485 B.C.) consulted, and Ctesias of Cnidus, personal physician to Artaxerxes II Mnemon (*regnabat* 405–359).[18] Later, according to a well-known passage in the *Dēnkart*, Shāpūr I, son of Ardashīr (*regnabat* 241–72) is supposed to have collected books on 'medicine, astronomy, motion, time, space, substance, creation, genesis, passing away, change and growth, and other arts and crafts' from India, the Byzantine empire and other countries.[11] This information is probably connected with the victory of

Shāpūr over the emperor Valerian in the year 260, when Valerian was captured and Roman technicians and scholars came into the country as prisoners, along with his army. They settled chiefly in Khūzistān, and the founding of the town Gondēshāpūr resulted from the attempt by the great king to prepare a home for the scholars so that their knowledge could benefit the country. Under Khosrau I Anōsharwān (*regnabat* 531–78), the empire of the Sasanids reached the peak of its cultural flowering. Paulus Persa dedicated his book on Aristotelian logic, written in Syriac, to this ruler. Greek influence can be clearly seen in the medical writings of the time: the concepts of cold, heat, dryness and wetness, were borrowed but polarized according to the dualist teaching of the Zoroastrians: cold and dryness are the evils which the doctor must combat by means of warm and wet medicaments and diet.[20] Although direct witnesses are almost completely lacking, one can assume with certainty that at the latest in the time of Khosrau I, complete Greek medical works were translated into Pahlavi. This conclusion is obvious from the whole cultural context. Sasanid art was influenced and moulded in numerous ways by Byzantine art.[21] There were middle-Persian translations of the agricultural work of Cassianus Bassus Scholasticus (sixth century A.D.), the astrological works of Vettius Valens (second century A.D.) and of Teucrus (second century B.C. or first century A.D.?)[22] as well as of the *Almagest* of Ptolemy.[23] From these we learn that their Persian versions were further translated into Arabic towards the end of the eighth or in the ninth century. From Arabic sources we can now work back to middle-Persian medical texts and I will try in what follows to present four works which were translated into Arabic.

The first work consists of a list of *Succedanea* (Ar. *abdāl al-adwiya*). In it is shown what drugs the apothecary may use as substitute when he cannot provide or procure those prescribed by the doctor for the patient. Such lists are well-known from antiquity. For example, a book *Peri antemballomenōn* is attributed to Galen. The little booklet here discussed, preserved only in its Arabic version, immediately reveals its Iranian origin because it uses almost exclusively ancient Persian names for plants and drugs. The white bryony (*Bryonia alba*) is called *hazār jashān* (instead of the Arabic *karma bayḍā'*), the dwarf laurel (*Daphne mezereum*) is *haft barg* (instead of *māzaryūn*), and the black nightshade (*Solanum nigrum*) is *rūbāh-turbak* (instead of *'inab ath-tha'lab*). The name of the author is Badīghūras in its Arabic form and it appears he was a Greek doctor named Pythagoras, employed, as once Democedes and Ctesias were, by the Persians; at least he was not earlier than the Sasanid period and therefore he may have worked in Gondēshāpūr. The Persians had assimilated his name into their language when it must have sounded Padhīghoras, which, when his writing was translated, was turned by the Arabs into Badīghūras.[24]

Of the second work about twenty-five fragments are preserved in Arabic authors.[25] From these it can be seen that the book had as its subject 'simple remedies'. It deals partly with drugs originating in India and unknown to the Greeks, as for example, marsh nut (*Semecarpus anacardium*, Ar. *balādhur*, from Pahlavi *balātur*, Sanskr. *bhallātaka*) and banana (*Musa paradisiaca*, Ar. *mawz*, for Pahlavi *mōz*, Sanskr. *mocā*). On the other hand, from time to time the degree of the effectiveness of the drugs is mentioned, and this is typical of Galen. The book must therefore have arisen where the lines of transmission from India and Greece intersected and this was presumably Sasanid Iran. On this supposition the name of the author can also be explained. In Arabic it reads al-Qulhumān or al-Qahlamān. It is formed like the Persian Pahlawān, Qahramān, Bahtakān or Marzubān (Marzpān). There are also parallels for the fact that Persian names, when used by the Arabs, were provided with the article: the Persian general taken prisoner by the Arabs in 642 at Shushtar was called by them al-Hurmuzān.

Things seem to have been similar in the case of a work quoted by ar-Rāzī under the title *The Old Medicine* (*aṭ-Ṭibb al-qadīm*).[26] By this is not meant, as one might at first suppose, the Hippocratic writing *De prisca medicina*; rather we find here an outline of general medicine dealing with facial paralysis, headaches, trachoma, dysentery, hysterical choking and other illnesses. It all corresponds exactly to the usual list of illnesses in Greek books. But here too, Indian drugs are mentioned so that once again one has to look for the origin of the book in Iran. After it was translated into Arabic, the title page apparently went missing so that ar-Rāzī could only refer to it under

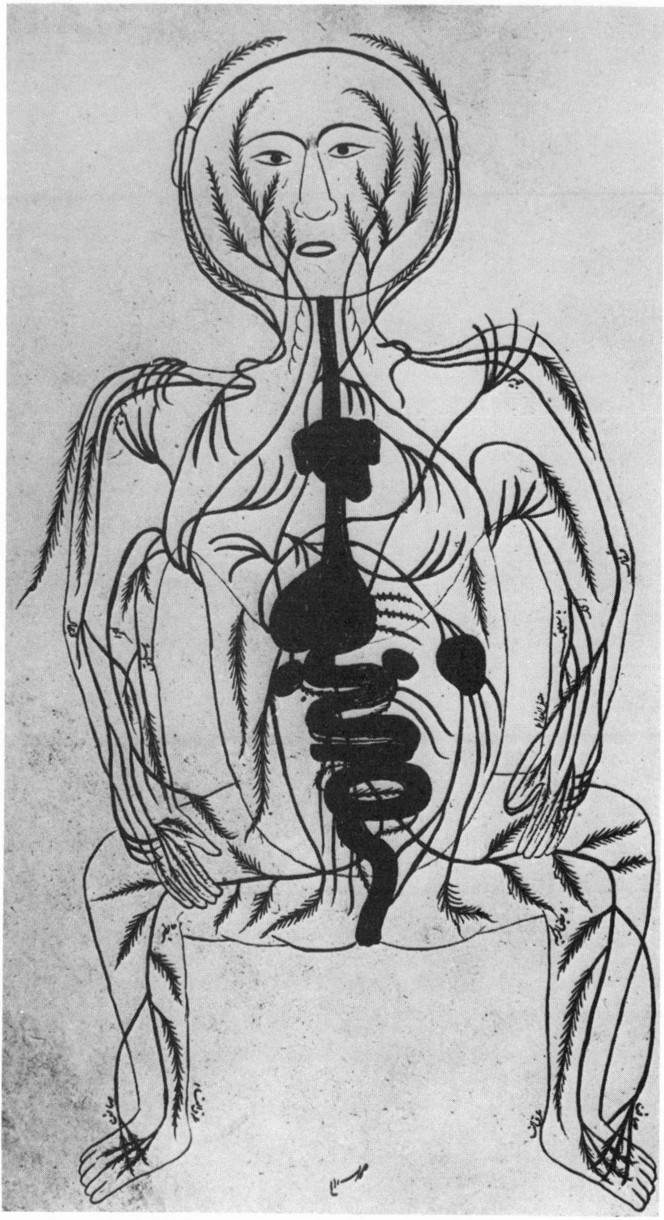

PLATE I. System of the veins, according to a Persian MS

كتب القانون في الطب

لابو علي الشيخ الرييس

ابن سينا

مع بعض تاليفه وهو علم المنطق وعلم الطبيعي
وعلم الكلام

ROMAE,
In Typographia Medicea.
M.D.XCIII.
Cum licentia Superiorum.

PLATE 2. Title-page of the *Canon of Medicine* by Avicenna, printed in Arabic type in Rome 1593

the provisional title of *The Old Medicine*.

The fourth work, however, does not appear to have been originally composed in Iran but to have taken the same course as the agricultural work of Cassianus and the *Astrologumena*. It is written in Greek and thence transmitted to the Arabs through Pahlavi. Its author was Xenocrates of Aphrodisias who lived about A.D. 70 and who recommended cures based on sympathetic magic using parts of organs, secretions and secreta from men and animals.[27] Galen wrote strong polemics against his unappetizing 'filth pharmacy'. We meet it all again in Arabic under the name of *Aṭ'hūrusfus*: 'If you take old, stale urine from a human being and let it trickle into the ear of someone with earache, it will be beneficial';[28] and 'if one takes a piece of ivory from a tusk and wraps it in a black cloth and hangs it round the necks of the cows, it will protect them against the plague (*wabā*)'.[29] But the name *Aṭ'hūrusfus* with this combination of sounds cannot be explained from either Greek or Arabic. It is however possible that the name of Xenocrates, because of the inadequacy of middle-Persian writing, became corrupted in this way.

Indian works

Because of its favoured geographical position, Persia took much from Indian medicine. Under Khosrau I, the Persian doctor Burzōē, whose autobiographical account has often been discussed,[30] travelled to India whence he brought back to his home not only the *Pancatantra* but also medical books. It appears that one of these books is still preserved in a medieval Greek translation[31] which might have emanated from an Arabic intermediate translation. Later, in the ninth century, the Arabs got to know a number of other Indian works. At that time Indian doctors were also practising at the caliph's court, but whether they alone were responsible for the transmission of those books is questionable. The *Caraka-Saṃhitā*, a medical compendium that contains the teachings of Āgniveśa,[32] was, according to the account by Ibn-an-Nadīm, first translated from the Indian into Persian and then translated further into Arabic by a certain ʿAbd-Allāh ibn-ʿAlī. The book was frequently used by Muḥammad ibn-Zakariyyā' ar-Rāzī, who quoted it by the term *Sharak*. Suśruta lived about A.D. 400. His manual, the *Suśruta-Saṃhitā*, belongs to the most significant Indian works. Ibn-an-Nadīm tells how the Barmakid Yaḥyā ibn-Khālid commissioned the Indian doctor, Mankah, to translate it. The same Mankah is also supposed to have translated the 'Book of Poisons of Shānāq'. This work is a very curious case. Cāṇakya, the minister of the king Candragupta of the dynasty of Mawrya (*c.* 320 B.C.), is designated in Arabic by Shānāq. He is the presumed author of a manual on the art of government, the *Kawṭiliyya Arthaśāstra*, but this work is only one of many sources of the book of poisons. Parallels in the contents are also found in Caraka and Suśruta, but the immediate Indian source of the 'book of poisons' is still unknown. This *Kitāb as-Sumūm* is at any rate the only Indian medical work of which the Arabic version is preserved completely even to-day in numerous manuscripts. By means of this book, a ruler is placed in the position of being able to protect himself against being poisoned.[33] In this connection we must also mention that a Persian-Arabic doctor, 'Alī ibn-Sahl aṭ-Ṭabarī, in the appendix to his *Kitāb Firdaws al-ḥikma* (published 850) has given an exposé of the system of Indian medicine. 'Alī has in this relied on the Persian or Arabic translations of the books of Caraka, Suśruta, Vāgbhata and Mādhavakara. The five elements, air, wind, fire, earth and water, are understood there not as material but as dynamic functional magnitudes. Instead of four there are only three humours (*doṣas*): wind, bile, and phlegm; and the seven elementary substances (*dhātus*) involved in digestion are blood, flesh, fat, bones, marrow and semen. But 'Alī ibn-Sahl did not identify himself with these teachings; he only described them. The main part of his book consists completely of the medicine of Hippocrates and Galen and the philosophy of Aristotle.[34]

The consequences

After this survey of material, let us pause to remind ourselves of the situation in which Arab doctors found themselves towards the end of the ninth century. As we have seen, the Arabs were influenced from four sides: by the Greeks, the Syrians, the Persians and the Indians. In this, the role of transmitting the Greek or Indian legacy fell chiefly to the Syrians and Persians. The most important component in both scope and content in this process of transmission was Greek medicine. We shall sketch briefly its development so that we can judge how the Arabs reacted and had to react to it.

The classical Greek medicine had taken an extraordinarily lively, varied and dramatic line of development. Already in the *Corpus hippocraticum* the different views of the schools of Cos and Cnidus were united. The book *De prisca medicina* was a programmatic work which was supposed to show the advantages of the 'old medicine' over the new philosophies. In *De natura hominis* the teaching about the humours in the sense of the scheme of four, is expanded and systematized. The Attic medicine was centred on the Peripatetics, but Diocles of Carystus had a special position. In Hellenistic times the great doctors, Erasistratus of Ceus and Herophilus of Chalcedon, broke away from humoral pathology. Praxagoras of Cos (*c.* 325 B.C.) is indeed a humoral pathologist but represented a doctrine of ten or eleven humours. The Methodists Asclepiades of Bithynia, Themison of Laodicaea and Soranus of Ephesus teach that illnesses depend on the different tensions in the pores. The medicine of the imperial period represented by Rufus, Galen and Aretaeus of Cappadocia, introduces a renaissance of Hippocratism but also eclectically includes the discoveries and ideas of Hellenistic medicine. Through the universal recognition of Galen, who saw in Hippocrates his great exemplar and the founder of scientific medicine generally, the humoral pathology gains the victory. Byzantine medicine consolidated Galenism. Certainly individual doctors, for example, Posidonius (fourth century) or Alexander of Tralles, bring completely new thoughts and information but there are no more new systems. What has been handed down was collected in large Summas and encyclopedias, like that of Oribasius above all, or the material was gathered in compendia. Thus, from the third century, the main element was Galenism.

Galen's medicine was markedly eclectic. In general physiology he had, as we have said, elaborated the doctrine of the humours; in special physiology he had used Platonic,[35] Stoic, and Peripatetic ideas; his anatomy was taken over from the Alexandrians, and in pharmacology he is specially indebted to

Dioscurides.[36] This eclecticism was further overlaid by the Arabs. The Arabs drew not only on Galen but also on other Greek doctors, in part directly from Hippocrates; after that, in dietetic questions, from Rufus of Ephesus, and through the Byzantine compilers (for example, Oribasius, Paul of Aegina) they got to know, at least in excerpt, the teachings of many other doctors. Thus they took over syndromes of illnesses lacking in Galen, such as lycanthropy from Aetius of Amida, who in this case reproduces what Marcellus of Side had maintained. While Galen took up a very reserved position as regards the practice of magic in medical treatment, Alexander of Tralles allows free rein to these irrational tendencies, and the translation of the work of Alexander had its effect on the Arabs. To the Hellenistic magic that he transmitted according to the *Physiologus* and the *Koiranides*, ʿAlī ibn-Sahl aṭ-Ṭabarī united the magic ideas and practices of his native Ṭabaristān. The knowledge of the bedouin Arabs, on the other hand, played only a small role: only ʿArīb ibn-Saʿīd al-Qurṭubī occasionally quotes bedouin sayings about the process of birth. But Arab folk-practices disguised as Ḥadīth of the Prophet, are collected together as 'prophetic medicine' and then mingled with Greek teachings. Dioscurides reigns supreme in materia medica, but early on, many new drugs came from Persia and India.

Arabic medicine offers therefore a very colourful and varied picture. There was no lack of outside stimulus, and one wonders whether this might not have led to a lively argument with Galenism, and whether Galen's doctrine might not have been severely tested or even revised. There were indeed some cases in which individual doctrines of Galen were criticized, but there was no revision, far less dissolution, of the general Galenic system. This could not happen because the lively development which classical Greek medicine had undergone came to a halt after the imperial period. This halt in development came to an end in the West only in Renaissance times when things started moving again through Vesalius and Paracelsus. Arabic medicine falls in the period of the medieval quiescence, though this must not be looked on as stagnation. The Arabs had received Greek medicine at the last stage of its development and they could do no other than assume that this system was perfect and final. When on occasion al-Majūsī reports on non-Galenic theories, he does so only to refute them at once, not to introduce a genuine, fruitful discussion in which justice is done to the other standpoint also. At one place[37] al-Majūsī reports that some philosophers assume not four elements but a single element, which according to some is the atom, to others the air, and again to others, water. At another place,[38] he informs us that according to some, the body consists not of four humours but only of one, for example, of blood. At a third place,[39] he quotes divergent teachings about the psychic pneuma: 'some scholars assert that this pneuma, which is located in the brain, is the soul, and that the soul is a body. Other people say that the pneuma is the tool of the soul, that it is used by all senses and that the soul is not a body...'. But these divergent teachings are for al-Majūsī, up to a point, only curiosities, and their representatives, whose names do not even deserve mention, are not people to be taken seriously.

Sometimes the differences in the teachings of the ancient doctors were registered factually: Aḥmad ibn-Muḥammad ibn-Yaḥyā al-Baladī tells in his book about children's diseases, how Galen completely forbade children to take wine, while Rufus allowed it in moderation.[40] In the same book (III, 7), he recounts how Hippocrates reckons sleeplessness among children's illnesses but that Galen is of a different opinion. ʿAlī ibn-Riḍwān asserts that in his commentary on the Hippocratic writing *De morbis muliebribus*, Asclepius contradicts Galen. But in no case does a creative argument with Galen arise.

It has therefore been asked whether the Arabs showed any originality: 'In speaking of Arab achievements in science and philosophy the important question to ask is: how far were the Arabs mere transmitters of what the Greeks had discovered and how far did they make original contributions?'[41] This does not seem to me to be a right question to ask because it applies to a period in which the question of originality does not arise, a period which was dominated by a scientific conception entirely different from our own. In the Islamic Middle Ages there was no real scientific research and there was no desire for empirical knowledge of reality. Thus, the doctor too, when dealing with the phenomenon of illness was not trying to discover new knowledge, or to reinterpret the processes which go on in the human body, or to develop new and more adequate therapies. For him, the literature of the ancients is both example and authority; he believes that in it a certain natural truth is laid down which he can only think about, develop, and comment on. His standpoint in regard to antiquity is not critical or reflective but naïve and accepting. Tradition is for him a treasure chest which he willingly makes use of, and in no way is it possible for him to experience it as a burden that he could or would shake off. He repeats the thoughts of the Greeks and collects and amasses what has been handed down. This effort reaches its peak in the encyclopedias, those great compendia of medicine left us by ar-Rāzī, al-Majūsī, az-Zahrāwī, Ibn-Sīnā and others. What they offer is not factual material extracted through observation, or through systematic research and experiments, but a construction based on theories. These theories were once formed by the Hippocratics and the Alexandrian doctors right down to Galen in the area of tension between philosophical theorems and the appearances of the healthy and unhealthy human organism. They are therefore genuine science. But since late antiquity and throughout the Middle Ages, man's attempts to observe nature herself were very weak. The prescribed thought-world is no longer corrected by appearances; the formation of concepts has ceased. New theses or systems can no longer be set up.

In what follows, we will try to make clear by some examples, what problems were bound up for the Arabs with the assimilation of Greek medicine.

Erratic blocks

When cultures meet and manifest themselves in great translating activity, it is customary to differentiate between two phases: one of reception, and one of assimilation. In the phase of reception, which precedes in time, the foreign books are at first only translated; later, in the phase of assimilation, the translated texts themselves are independently worked into new books. But reception and assimilation may also occur at the same time and in one person; for example, Ḥunayn translated many Greek books, but at the same time he wrote Arabic text-books for students and composed independent books about ophthalmology, dentistry or dietetics, the material for which he owed to Galen, Paul of Aegina, and others.

It sometimes happened that certain material was received but not assimilated. It never got beyond the reception stage although it was always repeated in the later literature of the Arabs. So it is, for instance, with the list of poisonous snakes which we know from the work entitled *De venenatis animalibus eorumque remediis* of Philumenus (*c.* third century A.D.). This list was presumably translated into Arabic from a pseudo-Galenic book on poisons whose author had taken it from Philumenus.[42] The translator, however, was unable to identify the thirty or so Greek snake-names and to match them with Arabic species. The Arabs had never distinguished so many species; in their language they possessed only a few general names for snakes, like *ḥayya*, *af'ā*, *thu'bān*, *raqshā*, and *shujā*. Moreover, many species of snake described by Philumenus could not possibly have occurred in Syria, Egypt and the Arabian peninsula, whereas other snakes were common to these countries which Philumenus could not have known. The translator of the Greek book of poisons has simply transliterated half of the Greek snake names. Thus *basiliskos* became *bāsilīqūs*, *mygalē* became *mūghālī* etc. He Arabized the other half of the names by loan renderings so that *khelidonia* became *khuṭṭāf*, *ptyas* became *bazzāqa*, *dipsas* became *mu'aṭṭisha* and *amphisbaina* became *ṭaffāra ilā l-jihatayn*. These loan renderings were for an Arab doctor just as meaningless as the transcriptions. In spite of this, this list of snakes with its descriptions of the appearance of the reptiles, the symptoms of the bites and the directions for treatment continued to be handed down. They are found as an erratic block in Avicenna, Ibn-Hubal, Najīb-ad-Dīn as-Samarqandī, Maḥmūd ibn-Ilyās ash-Shīrāzī and Ibn-al-Quff.[43]

A similar erratic block was probably the information about medicinal earths. Dioscurides[44] and Galen[45] enumerate the sigillated earth of Lemnus, a reddish clay stamped into pellets with the sacred seal of Artemis, the Samian earth, the earth of Chius, the Cimolean earth, the Armenian earth and other earths which were taken as remedies and in part were said to have achieved wonderful results. The *terra sigillata* was said to be good against lethal poisons and the bite of a mad dog, and the Armenian earth is the favourite remedy against plague. These earths confront us again in all Arab pharmacopias, in al-Majūsī (II, 130), Ibn-Sīnā[46] and in Ibn-al-Bayṭār from Malaga.[47] But what Arab apothecary in Spain, in Yemen or in Persia, would have been able to procure earths from the Aegean islands? In this instance too, dead book knowledge was conscientiously passed on through centuries.[48]

So it was too, in the case of some illness syndromes. The werwolf legend was indigenous in Arcadia. It was believed that men could from time to time transform themselves into wolves, who then performed their mischief. The doctor Marcellus of Side may have suspected that a psychopathological phenomenon lay concealed in this legend and so he subsumed the appearance of the werwolf as 'lycanthropy' among the mental illnesses. It was from him that Aetius of Amida took over lycanthropy and it reached the Arabs through the translation of his book, and al-Majūsī, Avicenna, az-Zahrāwī and others described it as a special form of melancholy under the name *quṭrub* just as Aetius had done. But no Arab doctor has ever in the course of his practice seen a werwolf!

Finally, we must mention a fourth example: in the numerous Greek treatises on hygiene, physical exercises are demanded, but these presuppose institutions like the gymnasium or the palaestra. The Arab authors demand the same gymnastic exercises, sometimes described in great detail, but in the Islamic town there was neither palaestra nor gymnasium. Gymnastics could not be practised! In spite of this, medical books always describe physical exercise at great length. On the other hand, when the writers on hygiene demanded that the baths be visited, this could be followed in Islamic countries because the ancient baths are faithfully copied and remain in use as 'Turkish baths' right up to the present day.[49]

I do not want to be misunderstood: naturally the rich medical literature of the Greeks gave the Arabs an immense stimulus and put them in a position to approach disease on an entirely new basis. But one must not forget that this was chiefly a matter of book knowledge, and this fact has come to be clearly seen by the way in which even a dead letter was handed down, often in comical fashion, and so preserved for centuries.

The elaboration of a scientific terminology

The translators who had to translate the Greek, Syrian, and Persian medical works into Arabic were confronted with the task of creating a technical terminology in Arabic for the new concepts and subjects. In so doing, as is everywhere the case, they have followed three methods: either they have taken over unchanged, the Greek, Syriac or Persian expressions as foreign words; or they have Arabized the foreign words with loan renderings; or thirdly, they have used old Arabic words in a terminologically restricted sense. The Greek *synokhos* (*pyretos*), 'unintermittent fever', is translated by *sūnūkhus*, *hēmitritaios*, 'semi-tertian fever', by *amiṭrīṭāwus*, *ēpialos*, 'ague', by *ībiyālūs*. *Ho lēthargos*, 'the lethargy', is transcribed *lītharghus*. Sometimes foreign words and integrated forms remain side by side; *to xērion*, 'desiccative powder', becomes in Syriac *ksīrīn* and in Arabic *iksīrīn*. Alongside this appears the form (*al-*)*iksīr* assimilated to the Arabic morpheme *if'īl*, and this was later to become our 'elixir'. We can see mirrored in the foreign words, as this example shows, the lines of transmission of ancient medicine sketched above: the Greek *kardamōmon*, 'cardamom', found its way into Arabic not in its original form but in the form *qurdamānā* which goes back to the Syriac, and the Greek *sagapēnon*, 'ferula persica', was known to the Arabs only in the middle-Persian form *sakbīnaj*.

Loan renderings are commonest. *Karkinos* 'cancer', became *saraṭān*; *alōpekia*, 'fox sickness', and *ophiasis*, 'snake sickness', both denoting loss of hair, became *dā' ath-tha'lab* and *dā' al-ḥayya*. *Hē hierā nūsos*, 'the sacred disease', a name for epilepsy, was reproduced in Arabic by *al-maraḍ al-ilāhī*, 'the divine disease', or *al-maraḍ al-kāhinī*, 'the diviner's disease'.[50] In the case of the skins of the eyes, we find the rendering *epipephykōs khitōn* corresponds to *aṭ-ṭabaqa al-multaḥima*; *keratoeidēs khitōn* to *aṭ-ṭabaqa al-qarniyya*; *sklēros khitōn* to *aṭ-ṭabaqa aṣ-ṣulba*; *amphiblēstroeidēs khitōn* to *aṭ-ṭabaqa ash-shabakiyya* etc. Numerous plant-names are formed in this way: *ho potamogeitōn*, 'the pondweed', became *jār an-nahr*; *mēkōn aphrōdēs*, 'opium poppy', became *khashkhāsh ẓabadī*. In the case of binary naming, there are hybrids made out of foreign words and loan renderings: *lykhnis stephanōmatikē*, 'rose campion', became *likhnīs al-iklīliyya*; *hē dysenteria hēpatītis*, 'dysentery arising from the liver' became *ad-dusanṭāriyā al-kabadiyya*. Sometimes such forms have come about by wrong translation: the Greek plural *hai khoirades*, 'scrofulous swellings in the glands of the neck', becomes in Arabic *al-khanāzīr*, 'the pigs', because the word was confused with *hoi khoiroi*, 'the pigs'. The *pneuma zōtikon* 'the vital spirit', is in Arabic *rūḥ ḥayawānī*, 'animal spirit', because the adjective *zōtikos*, 'vital', was confused with *zōōdēs*, 'like an animal'.

The third possibility, the use of existing Arabic words in a specific meaning, is less common. *Kalaf* was originally in Arabic a general term for 'reddish-brown colour'. The doctors used this word to denote the Greek *ephēlis*, a skin infection characterized by an abnormally dark pigmentation. *Ramad* was originally eye inflammation in general. It was then used by the doctors as the equivalent of *ophthalmia*, 'trachoma'. *Iklīl* means in general 'crown'. In the translation of Dioscurides, it is used to denote the Greek *skiadeion*, 'umbel'.[51] In classical Arabic, the cerebral membrane is denoted by *umm ad-dimāgh*, 'mother of the brain'. But the translators of Galen learnt that there are two cerebral membranes, a thick outer one (*hē pakheia mēninx*) and a thin, inner one (*hē leptē mēninx*). As a result, they took over only the first half of the expression and added to it the different attributes 'hard' and 'thin' and talked of *al-umm al-jāfī* and *al-umm ar-raqīq*. When Constantinus Africanus (d. 1087) translated the *Kitāb al-Malakī* of 'Alī ibn-al-'Abbās al-Majūsī into Latin, he translated *al-umm al-jāfī* by *dura mater* and *al-umm ar-raqīq* by *pia mater*. In so doing, he extracted the wrong meaning from the adjective *raqīq*, which can mean tender, frail, weak, delicate, as well as loving, affectionate. Both expressions are still used to-day in modern anatomy.[52] The Greek *kollyrion* is used to denote 'eye-salve' as well as 'suppository', 'pessary', an equivocation which could lead to dangerous confusion in pharmacy. The Arabic translators failed to take the opportunity to purify the nomenclature and in faithful imitation of the Greeks, have denoted both types of prescription by *shiyāf*.

In many cases they in no way succeeded in creating a clear, universal nomenclature. So it was with phrenitis, the name of an illness that can be most closely identified with our meningitis.[53] The Greek word *phrenītis* came into Arabic as a foreign word in the form *farānīṭis*, but the diacritical point of the first letter soon became corrupted so that many doctors, including Ibn-Sīnā, have written and pronounced it *qarānīṭis*. As the word has also been entered in alphabetically arranged glossaries under *Qāf*, this form may not be 'emended'. When the *Qānūn* of Ibn-Sīnā was eventually translated into Latin, the letter 'n' too was wrongly pointed so that the word sounded *karabitus* in Latin.[54] But early on, a Persian word was used for phrenitis. In the translations of the *Aphorisms* of Hippocrates (VI, 11; VII, 12), of the *Testament* of Hippocrates and the manuals of Alexander of Tralles (I, 509 ff.), and of Paul of Aegina,[55] *birsām* constantly stands for *phrenītis*. This is derived from the Pahlavi *war* (breast) and *sām* (inflammation) and so really means 'breast inflammation' or 'pleurisy'. In this case there must have been originally a confusion with the word *sarsām*, 'head inflammation',[56] and this confusion must have arisen because the word *barsām* or *birsām* had already found its way into pre-Islamic Arabic poetry and become frequent there.[57] In some texts *sirsām* and *birsām* are mentioned one after the other.[58] Their authors have understood these two words to mean two different illnesses. But in the case of ar-Rāzī and other doctors, *birsām* and *sirsām* are used as being fully synonymous and interchangeable. Ar-Rāzī (Ḥāwī, XV, 65) differentiates only in so far as he writes that the 'people' or the uninitiated (*al-'āmma*) would say *birsām*, while the doctors would use *sirsām*. In another place (Ḥāwī, I, 219), he says, however, that the expression *birsām* is used for two illnesses, for the *shawṣa* (by which is meant a sort of pleurisy) as well as for meningitis and the latter is *sirsām*. Ibn-Sīnā (Qānūn, I, 302 ff.), a Persian from birth like ar-Rāzī, bemoans the confusion of language: people who knew nothing about languages, would also use *birsām* to denote phrenitis, yet *birsām* is of Persian origin and *bar* meant 'breast' and *sām*, 'inflammation, disease'; the word for 'head', on the other hand, was *sar*. Al-Jāwālīqī (d. 1144) writes similarly in his *Dictionary of Foreign Words*.[59] But al-Jāwālīqī recognizes, as do the philologists Ibn-Durayd, Abu-Naṣr al-Bāhilī and as-Sukkarī, the genuine Arabic word *mūm* as an equivalent for *birsām*, and Ibn-Durayd, just to complete the confusion, says somewhere else[60] that the Persian word *birsām* is a popular expression and that one must on the other hand say *jirsām* or *jilsām* in the classical language. Finally, among the doctors each has his own opinion; al-Majūsī (I, 327) teaches that *sirsām* has its origin in a hot dyscrasy in the brain itself or in a hot swelling in the cerebral membrane, that *birsām* likewise arises in the brain but is due to a swelling in the spleen, which is connected with the brain by a nerve track. But *sirsām* denotes not only phrenitis but also lethargy, and a distinction is made between these two illnesses by calling phrenitis 'the hot meningitis' (*as-sirsām al-ḥārr*) and lethargy 'the cold meningitis' (*as-sirsām al-bārid*).[61] It was therefore no easy matter for students of Arabic medicine to find their way about in the maze of very varied terminology.

The Islamization of certain Greek tenets

A further problem was tied up with the take-over of Greek-Hellenistic medicine by the Arabs: Greek medicine, which had originated in the sphere of Greek religion, now had to come to terms with the Islamic religion which knew no mythological gods but only the One God. Asclepius was the god of healing and the Asclepieia were places of healing and worship at the same time. Whereas in an outline of medical history, Asclepius played the role of god among the Greeks, among the Muslims he was only honoured as the discoverer and originator of medicine; in other words, he was taken out of myth and placed in history, which as a result received fantastic chronological features. This historicizing of Asclepius meant that when the Hippocratic oath was translated, he alone of the Greek gods and goddesses mentioned there, was tolerated and could survive. The Greek oath begins with the words: 'I swear by Apollo Physician and Asclepius and Hygieia and Panaceia and all the gods and goddesses, making them my witnesses, that I will fulfil according to my ability and judgement this oath and this covenant'.[62] In Arabic, on the other hand, it runs: 'I swear by God, Lord of life and death, the giver of health and the creator of healing and every therapy, and I swear by Asclepius and I swear by the saints of God, be they men or women, all together, and I appeal to them altogether as witnesses, that I shall stand by this oath and contract'. Other gods and demigods were simply changed. According to Galen,[63] the melancholic thinks that Atlas holds up the heavens but that he grows tired under the weight and that the heavens could then fall down. In the writings of Is'ḥāq ibn-ʿImrān about melancholy, God (*Allāh*) holds the heavens. But this makes the example absurd or blasphemous because a weakness of God is irreconcilable with the dogma of his omnipotence.

Certain problems arose too, through Islamic law. Oribasius[64] had recommended the sprinkling of an umbilical hernia in an infant with the ashes of the bones of a pig. But the pig is forbidden to Muslims. And so Ibn-al-Jazzār writes in his book on paediatrics[65] that one should take the ashes of the Achilles tendon of a calf. Rufus had written a book on the dietetic uses of wine, in which he even advises to give small children wine. But wine too is forbidden in Islam and so the book should not really have been translated at all. It says much for the liberal and realistic spirit of the time that despite this it was translated into Arabic and quoted from not only by the doctor ar-Rāzī but also by the literary author, ar-Raqīq an-Nadīm al-Qayrawānī (*c.* 1000).[66]

The recovery of lost Greek texts

The great translation movement had, as mentioned, brought hundreds of Greek works to the Arabs. A fact is tied up with this which does not affect Islamic medical history but which is of the greatest importance for present-day philology and historiography, and which must not go unmentioned here. We must therefore take a look at the history of the transmission.

Galen's works are handed down chiefly in late manuscripts of the fifteenth century. In addition, the somewhat older Greco-Latin translations of Burgundio of Pisa (d. 1193),[67] Nicolas of Regium (1280–1350) and Peter of Abano (before 1303) are also significant: they have preserved for us some works of which the originals are lost. In view of this unfavourable state of the transmission, the Arabic versions are of the greatest importance: produced in the ninth century, they are based on Syriac or Greek manuscripts, which are at least six to seven centuries older than those preserved for us. As a result, considerable possibilities arise for the emending and editing of the Greek texts. But most important of all, numerous writings that were lost in the Greek remained preserved in Arabic dress. I shall give some examples of this.

Galen's chief anatomical work, *Peri anatomikōn egkheirēseōn*, consisted originally of fifteen books. In Greek, however, only books I–VIII and the beginning of book IX are extant. But the Arabic translation has preserved the complete text. Since Max Simon edited the Arabic texts of books IX–XV in 1906 and translated them into German, the complete work is accessible again to researchers. In the interval there has also been an English translation of the last seven books.[68]

Another, until recently unknown, anatomical treatise is the work about the differences of the homoeomeral parts of the body, *Peri tēs tōn homoiomerōn sōmatōn diaphorās*. Galen dedicated the work to the philosopher Antisthenes who had a lively interest in anatomy, and to whom he had dedicated two other treatises, namely, *De venarum arteriarumque dissectione* and *De nervorum dissectione*. Homoeomeral are, according to the teaching of Aristotle and also of Galen, such substances in themselves uniform and homogeneous, for example, metals, stones or wood, and also organic substances like flesh, skin or bones. Opposing them are the anhomoeomeral organs, for example, the extremities or the head. If one dissects these parts of the body, one eventually comes to homoeomeral substances, which can only be quantitatively separated. A bone can only be broken up into bone parts or splinters, but these particles show the same character as the whole bone. Galen enumerates about forty-five homoeomeral substances in his work, and these, to a certain extent, form the anatomical foundation stones of the human body. In so doing, he tries to ascertain the real anatomical facts and to avoid a classification which could be understood by the conventional use of language. Not everything that has its own name constitutes a separate species. The rediscovered text is also interesting from the point of view of medical history since the doctrine of the homoeomeral organs has dominated anatomy right down to the beginning of modern times and since it has stood in the way of histological research.[69]

Only two small Greek fragments remain of the work, *About Medical Experience*, *Peri tēs iatrikēs empeirias*, which Agostino

Gadaldini of Modena translated into Latin in the sixteenth century. An Arabic manuscript of Hagia Sophia in Istanbul, however, contains the complete text, which Richard Walzer published in Arabic and in an English translation in 1944.[70] Galen wrote this treatise before the year 150 in Pergamum when not yet 21 years old. It is supposed to reproduce the content of a disputation between the dogmatist Pelops, Galen's teacher, and the empiricist Philippus. In a long polemical speech, Philippus makes clear what is to be understood by the position held by the empirical school of thought. As the original writings of the empirical school were already lost in late antiquity, the new text is able to enrich our knowledge of that medical trend which had developed about 200 B.C. Its representatives got their experience at the sick bed and made the observation of successful treatment into a basic principle of medical research, rejecting as definite sceptics a theoretical/scientific basis for medicine.[71]

The work, *About the Examination of the Doctor* is not known to Greek texts even by title. Although Galen did not mention it in his self-bibliographies, that is, in the writings *De libris propriis* and *De ordine librorum suorum*, there is no doubt at all about its authenticity. Its Arabic translation is preserved in two manuscripts in Alexandria and Bursa, but not edited. The excerpts from it which were previously known give at least a first impression of its content. Since an examination and inspection of the doctor by the state authorities does not exist, it is left to the patient to examine the doctor of his choice. Galen now gives advice as to how the patient can decide on the ability and trustworthiness of the doctor by observing his life and successful results. In illustration he draws on all sorts of anecdotes from his own life and in his well-known boastful manner, does not hesitate to put his own excellence and superiority in a good light. In this way we learn a lot about Galen's biography. When in the new work he tells how, not yet 30 years old, he was on his return to Pergamum entrusted by the arch-priest with the office of physician to the gladiators, this detail, which is confirmed by other sources, is at the same time a criterion of the authenticity of the work.

As fifth example, I would like to draw attention to Galen's commentary on the Hippocratic work, *About the Atmosphere*

(*De aere aquis locis*), of which only four short passages are preserved in Greek, quoted anonymously by Oribasius. In the ninth century Ḥunayn ibn-Is'ḥāq translated this commentary into Syriac for Salmawayh ibn-Bunān, and Ḥubaysh translated the Syriac version into Arabic for Muḥammad ibn-Mūsā. In 1299 Salomon ben-Nathan Hameati translated the Arabic text into Hebrew, but all that is preserved is an incomplete manuscript in Oxford of this Hebrew version. Finally, the Hebrew version was translated into Latin by Moses Alatino. Thus, up to now, if one had wanted to use Galen's commentary, one had to resort to the fragmentary Latin version, accessible in an early printed edition; but this marks the end of a long tradition and understandably is extremely full of mistakes and very deformed. The Syriac text too, is, like the Greek, lost, and of the Arabic version for a long time only a few excerpts were known, that is, passages which ar-Rāzī, Ibn-Sīnā, ʿAlī ibn-Riḍwān, Maimonides and others had copied. It was a sensation for philologists when in 1971 it was announced that the complete Arabic version is preserved in a manuscript in the collection of Aḥmad Ṭalʿat Bey (d. 1927) in Cairo. Galen's commentary has therefore been recovered in a fairly early stage of the tradition. We now know that Galen also commented on the ethnographical parts of the Hippocratic work and that he sometimes marked the textual variants of Dioscurides and Artemidorus Capiton, thereby providing us with valuable criteria for the early textual history.

I could continue the list of Galenic writings which have been recovered only from the Arabic tradition, or which could be recovered, but I shall be content with these five examples and, instead, shall refer to another doctor, Rufus of Ephesus, in whose case the state of the tradition is similar. As mentioned already, fifty-eight of his writings were translated into Arabic in the ninth century, but only four remain in their entirety in Greek. However, Rufus was already considerably copied by Oribasius and Aetius, so that to these four manuscripts, a considerable number of Greek fragments can be added.

Up till now, the work of Rufus on jaundice, *Peri ikteru*, was known only through paragraphs 17 and 18 of Book x of Aetius. Aetius had there, in accordance with his usual custom as compiler, intermingled the work of Rufus and all that Galen

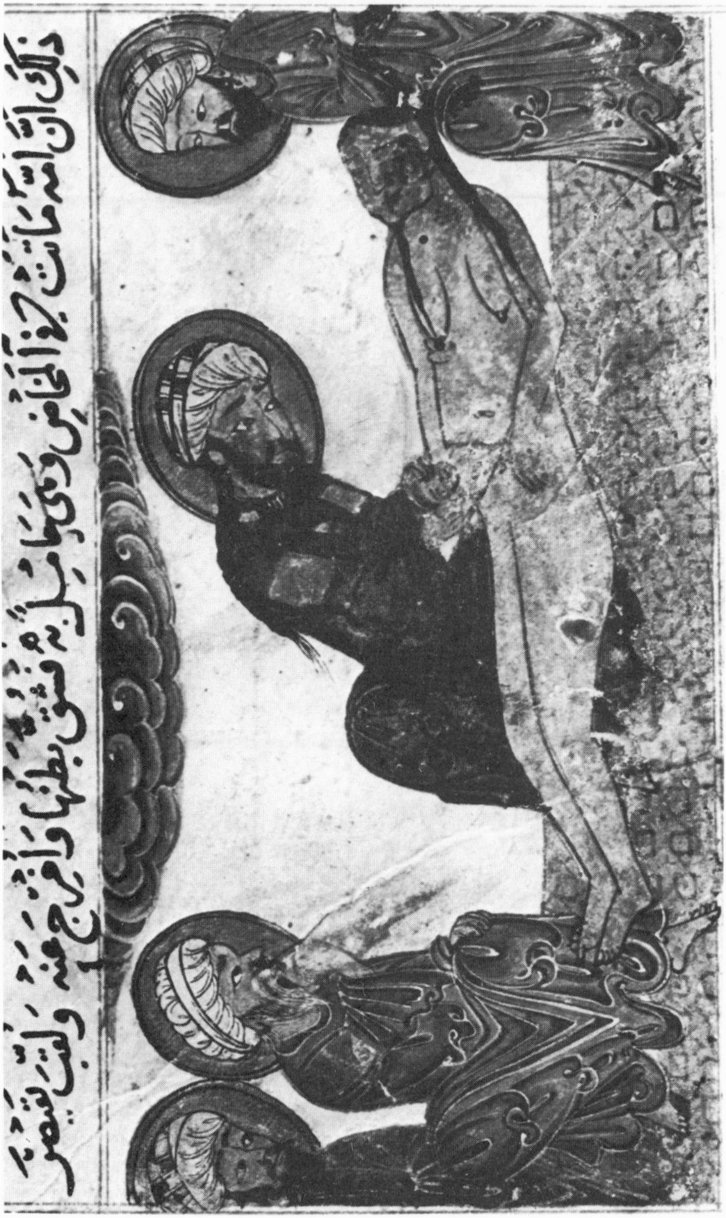

PLATE 3. Cesarian section, according to an Arabic MS

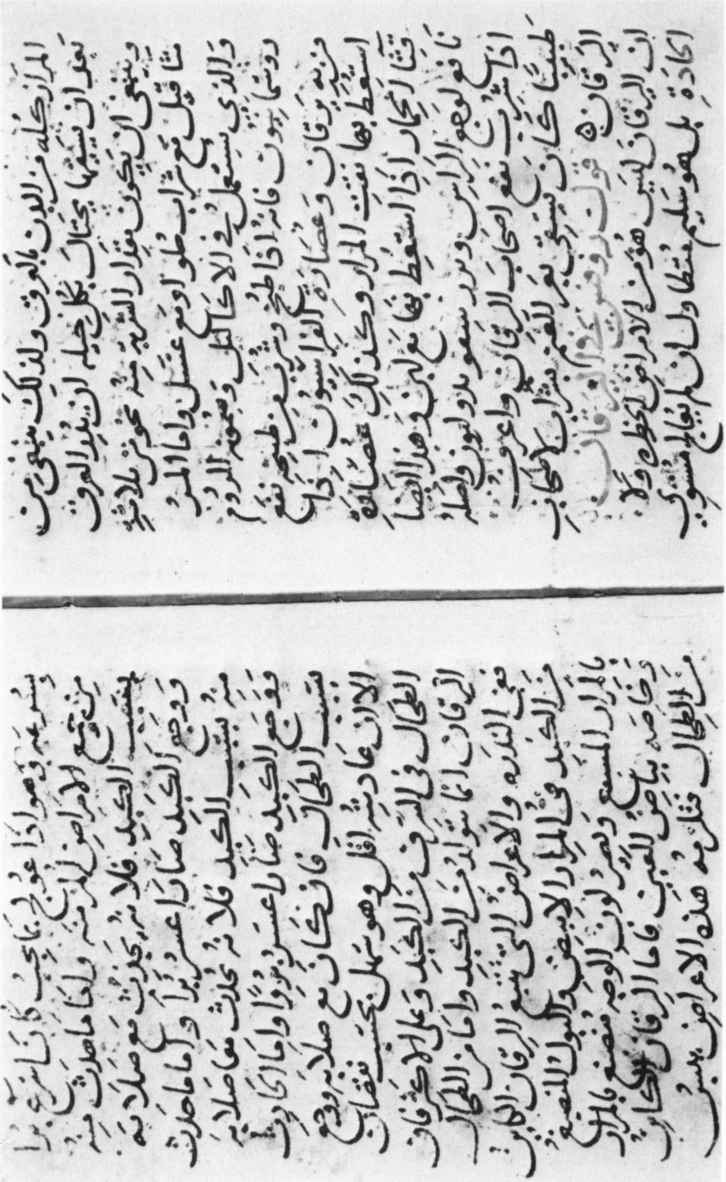

PLATE 4. Beginning of the tract on 'Jaundice' by Rufus of Ephesus, according to an Arabic MS

in his book, *De locis affectis*,[72] had written on jaundice, without distinguishing the individual contributions of the two authors. The passages by Rufus are now easily picked out because the complete text of his treatise is preserved in a manuscript in the Preussische Staatsbibliothek in Berlin. He begins with the words:

> Jaundice belongs neither to the dangerous, nor to the acute diseases; rather, it is benign but lengthy if not quickly treated. Given the required treatment, it can be cured more quickly than other chronic illnesses. That type which appears with the liver as basis is more difficult to heal, because hardness and pain occur simultaneously in the liver. On the other hand, the type that appears with the spleen for basis is easy to treat, even when accompanied by hardness and pain, because the spleen has a smaller compass than the liver. But generally, jaundice arises in the liver and seldom in the spleen.

The following description of the symptoms of the illness is distinguished by its precision and exactness:

> The symptoms which follow hepatic jaundice are white bile and urine saturated and coloured with bile. The face too, is coloured by bile, especially the whites of the eyes. The following symptoms occur in spleen jaundice: dryness of the body; the colour of the stools is not unusually white; urine tends to be black, indeed the whole body colour tends to be black. The whole is followed by twitching, loss of appetite and dislike of sweet foods. Those badly affected by this illness, suffer from sleeplessness, depression and restlessness, and they cannot perspire. Some patients perspire very slightly and lose a little bile with the perspiration. Others perspire many times in the bath. Finally there are those in whom bile comes out in the nasal mucus and in the secretion from the eyes.

Galen's details are more theoretically orientated: he discusses the various types of jaundice and its origin and argues from pathological and anatomical conditions which could cause a blockage of the liver. Rufus tackles the question in a more practical manner: he gives advice for a suitable diet and writes prescriptions of combined drugs. These procedures are very characteristic of both authors.

Rufus also wrote about loss of memory, *Peri mnēmēs apolōlyias*, a theme seldom touched upon in the psycho-pathological literature of the ancients. Once again it is Aetius who has combined Galen's expositions in *De locis affectis*[73] with the treatise of Rufus, but without marking the boundaries. But a longer extract from the Arabic translation of the work of Rufus transmitted by ar-Rāzī,[74] enables us to determine the boundary. We can immediately recognize the main conception of Rufus: cold and wet damage the memory, therefore one must use warming and drying means to effect an improvement but one must move forward gradually and step by step, because otherwise sudden extreme heat would do more harm than good. That children have an excellent memory, although their temperament is wet can be explained by the fact that their thinking is free from worries and the strain of study. For much study dries up the brain.

A third text is only preserved in an Arabic manuscript in the Bodleian Library in Oxford.[75] It consists of a collection of twenty-one clinical reports which are headed 'Examples and particular methods of treatment by Rufus'. As an example, I shall quote the text of the third case history. There Rufus writes:

> I know a man in whom melancholy began by the burning of the blood. The man was peaceful, and the fear and worry that had struck him were not severe, and what is more, both were a little mixed with joy. The cause of his illness was his constant brooding over the intricacies of geometry; he also took part in the social gatherings of the princes. Because of all these things, a pathological amount of black bile collected in him at a time when a man's age encourages the growth of melancholy anyway, I mean the time of decline; and added to this the fact that as a young man he had already had a quick temper. Now in advancing age, the black bile collected in him. Generally it afflicted him at night as a result of lying awake, and also at dawn. However, if he were asleep at dawn, he saw in his sleep, which alternated with a lethargy produced through sleeplessness, fleeting phantoms. Then he was treated by an inexperienced doctor. He emptied him and got him to vomit several times with sharp medicines but he failed to restore

> right balance to his temperament. The correcting of the temperament is, however, in this sort of illness the most important therapeutic measure, because it is the dyscrasy which produces such a humour and the production of the humour can only be ended by correcting the temperament. But after his temperament had become sharp by this medicine, the burning in his body increased and his case became worse to the extent of madness. He wanted neither to eat nor drink and eventually he died.

Now it is well known that Rufus wrote a book about melancholy[76] and in this book he assumes a direct connection between age and a disposition to melancholy. The older a man, the greater is the danger that he will become melancholic and it is precisely this theory that is brought out in this case history.

The book *De melancholia* is also lost in the Greek. For this reason, the fifteen quotations in the *Kitāb al-Ḥāwī* of ar-Rāzī are a modest but valuable substitute. But as evidence for Rufus, the *Treatise on Melancholy* published by Is'ḥāq ibn-'Imrān, personal physician to the Aghlabid sultan Ziyādat-Allāh III (*regnabat* 903–9) towards the end of his life, is perhaps just as important. Is'ḥāq begins his work with the words:

> I have read no satisfying book or comprehensive details about melancholy by any ancient author except one by a man among the ancients named Rufus of Ephesus. Now although this man has written a book in two chapters on this illness in which he has used his utmost intellectual endeavours and has conducted excellent investigations into the illness, its symptoms and the method of its treatment, he has nevertheless, despite all his ability, treated only one type of this illness, namely, hypochondria, and has omitted to mention the other types.

From this testimony and from the quotations which Is'ḥāq has incorporated in his work, we can gather that Rufus assumed a somatic cause for melancholy: when in the hypochondria or in the neighbourhood of the orifice of the stomach, following a disturbance of the digestion, a large amount of black bile collects, a black bile vapour rises from it into the brain, as the result of which, sadness, depression and hallucinations appear. But according to Is'ḥāq's interpretation, this is only one type of melancholy. He follows Galen who, in his work *De locis affectis*,[77] assumed three types of melancholy: in addition to the hypochondriac type there is a second, which causes the blood of the whole body to become black bile, and also a third, in which this black bile-blood is found only in the brain.

Ar-Rāzī has also preserved a few small fragments from the work *On the Upbringing of Children*, *Peri komidēs paidiu*; but considerably more numerous and comprehensive are the excerpts which Aḥmad ibn-Muḥammad al-Baladī (*c.* 990) has incorporated in his book, *Kitāb Tadbīr al-ḥabālā wa-l-aṭfāl*. After taking away the doublets, there remain eighteen Arabic fragments which complement most excellently the excerpts from Rufus's book which Oribasius transmitted. In Oribasius, only chapter 38 of the so-called *Libri incerti* has as headline the words: '*On the Upbringing of Children; from Rufus*', but the Arabic texts show by verbal correspondences that chapters 31, 42 and 43 also belong to Rufus's work. By comparing the Arabic with the Greek tradition, it has thus been possible to reconstruct Rufus's book in all essential points.[78] Rufus has accordingly written about the wet-nurse and the qualities she should possess, about the quality of her milk and how she should feed herself. Then he deals with children's complaints and has written about skin eruptions, teething, spasms, aphthae, bed-sores, ear and eye diseases, etc. On the care of infants, he mentions bathing and suitable feeding. One passage is particularly interesting in this connection and is found more fully and exactly in al-Baladī (II, 39) than in Oribasius:

> I praise the people called Lacedaemonians because they do not give their children enough to satisfy them completely. As a result, they are of good height and their bodies well-proportioned and they suffer no mishap like spasms, melancholy, fear, pain round the heart or anything else. If you want a child to grow tall and straight, with a good complexion, and not turned in on himself, avoid over-feeding him and follow the teaching of the Lacedaemonians and the qualities one can observe among them. For when a child is completely satisfied, it sleeps much and becomes lethargic, and its belly is distended and full of wind, and its urine watery.

We know the aims of Spartan feeding from the accounts by Xenophon and Plutarch. Plutarch says that bodies develop in stature when the pneuma is not checked by having to consume too much food. It can then rise easily and without hindrance and this makes the body slim and large. This tallies completely as to content with Rufus's presentation, but Rufus, unlike Plutarch, does not mention the pneuma. By so doing, he forgoes an explanation of the causal connection between nourishment and growth. A doctrine lies at the basis of this which is made explicit in the Hippocratic work, *De natura pueri*. There we read: 'Flesh is formed from the blood; but when it has increased, it is divided up by the pneuma so that like finds like, and as a result, individual members (limbs) form themselves out of the parts of the breathed-in pneuma.'

A second passage from the writing of Rufus about the upbringing of children is especially interesting. Rufus comments there on the question whether the enjoyment of wine should from a hygienic standpoint be permitted or forbidden to children. He argues from the concepts of heat and cold.

> The heat of children is, in relation to their wetness, not great. One can deduce this from the slackness, weakness and flabbiness of their bodies, and from the weakness of their voices. For all this does not appear in people in whom heat is dominant, but only in people of a cold constitution. But heat strengthens and firms the body, and keeps reason and insight together. It is therefore clear that children conceal much cold in them for their colour is white, their hair thin, they pass much urine, and their joints are tender.

Because wine increases the 'innate heat' in the body, children too, should be given wine to drink from time to time. Now Rufus had to establish this standpoint against the authority of Plato, who in his *Laws* strictly forbade children the pleasures of wine. In so doing, Rufus also differs from Galen who quotes the Platonic passage in his book *Quod animi mores corporis temperamenta sequantur* (ch. 10) and is in complete agreement with Plato. Wine is forbidden to children, Galen says, because by their very nature they are already warm and full-blooded.

Rufus, however, based his opinion in another work, the above-mentioned *Book of Wine*, which again we know only from an Arabic source, namely, the *Kitāb Quṭb as-surūr fī awṣāf al-khumūr*, composed by ar-Raqīq an-Nadīm al-Qayrawānī. Ar-Raqīq there quotes Rufus, who wrote as follows:

> The wonderful, special properties of wine are such that it benefits all mankind, of all ages, at all seasons and in all places. One should give infants and children as much as they can tolerate; more than that to adolescents, young men and men in their prime; but for old men there is nothing that will more advance their well-being and bodily health than wine, because they have a great need for what warms them. Children need a thing whose heat is advantageous for them because heat has not yet reached its full measure in them.[79]

We see that the information from the different sources forms a coherent picture.

What has been illustrated from Galen and Rufus here, can also be shown in the case of further Greek doctors, for example, Crito, Philagrius, Paulus, Magnus, and others. I have perhaps dwelt rather fully on these things. But it must be made clear that Arabic medicine can afford the greatest possible service to the classical philologists and medical historians of to-day. What happened in Baghdad in the ninth century, had its effect on the West in the eleventh and twelfth centuries, by providing it, through translations, with practical medicine, and again it has its repercussions for us in the twentieth century by opening up new sources for our historians.

THREE

SURVEY OF THE HISTORY OF ARABIC MEDICINE

In what follows the reader will be briefly made acquainted with the names of the most important Arab physicians.

ʿAlī ibn-Sahl Rabban aṭ-Ṭabarī was born about the year 810 in Merv as the son of a Christian scholar. He became secretary to the prince Māzyār ibn-Qārin in Tabaristan, the Persian province on the Caspian Sea, but after Māzyār's fall fled to Rayy. His *Kitāb Firdaws al-ḥikma* (*The Paradise of Wisdom*), one of the first compendia of medicine in Arabic, was completed in 850 and dedicated to the caliph al-Mutawakkil. It rests largely on Greek sources, on Hippocrates, Galen, Aristotle, Dioscurides and other authors, who are quoted by ʿAlī in a free adaptation of Syriac translations. In ʿAlī the intermingling of rational and magical observation of nature is specially marked, an attitude of mind which characterizes many medieval scholars. As an appendix to his book ʿAlī includes an exposition of the system of Indian medicine, a rare phenomenon in Arabic medieval literature. He drew his knowledge from the Persian or Arabic translations of the works of Caraka, Suśruta, Vāgbhata and Mādhavakara. In this way ʿAlī laid the foundations for a comprehensive study of two different medical systems, but this road was not followed by later authors.

Abū-Zakariyyā' Yūḥannā ibn-Māsawayh (*c.* 777–857) was said to have been commissioned by the caliph al-Ma'mūn to direct the activity of translation, but, as far as we know, produced no translations himself. As personal physician to the caliphs al-Ma'mūn, al-Muʿtaṣim, al-Wāthiq and al-Mutawakkil he spent nearly his whole life in Baghdad and Samarra. Among his pupils was for a while Ḥunayn ibn-Is'ḥāq, for whom he produced a small work of 132 aphorisms which in part show a close resemblance to the Hippocratic sayings (in the *Aphorisms* and in the work *De aere aquis locis*). Ibn-Māsawayh wrote a large work on general pathology, the *Kitāb al-Kamāl wa-t-tamām*, of which numerous fragments are preserved. Apart from this he dealt with many pathological and physiological questions in monographs.

Ḥunayn ibn-Is'ḥāq al-ʿIbādī (d. 873 or 877) has already (p. 9f. above) been assessed as translator of Greek works. He did not limit himself to pure reception, however, but independently composed many medical monographs. Especially well known was the *Kitāb al-Mudkhal fī ṭ-ṭibb*, an introductory manual in which the basic problems of general medicine were presented in diaeretic form, including pharmaceutics and uroscopy. In this Ḥunayn did not always start from Galen's original works (which contained contradictions and ambiguities) but rather made use of the late Alexandrian medicine with its synopses, which went beyond Galen in systematizing and schematizing the material. The Latin translation, which represents only the beginning of the fairly extensive work, bears the title *Isagoge in artem parvam Galeni*, but this is misleading because the original work of Ḥunayn goes far beyond the terms of reference of the *Ars parva*.

A work on ophthalmology exists, the *Kitāb al-ʿAshr maqālāt fī l-ʿayn*, which, as the title states, consists of ten articles that were written in the course of thirty years and then made into a book. It formed the starting-point for the important specialized ophthalmological literature produced by the Arabs, and has become known in two Latin versions under the misleading titles, *Galeni liber de oculis translatus a Demetrio* and *Liber de oculis Constantini Africani*.[1] Ḥunayn's treatise on dentistry, the *Qawl fī Ḥifẓ al-asnān wa-stiṣlāḥi-hā*, also appears to have been the first comprehensive presentation in its special field.[2]

Ḥunayn published his large book on diet, the *Kitāb al-Aghdhiya*, in both an Arabic and a Syriac version.[3] In it, as he says in the introduction, he has gathered together the teachings of Galen, Hippocrates, Dioscurides, Rufus, Phylotimus, Euryphon, Dieuches, Mnesitheus of Athens, Mnesitheus of Cyzicus, Diocles, Athenaeus from Attalia, Xenocrates and Antyllus. Some of these authors, however, he could quote only indirectly from Galen or Oribasius. The book comprises three parts. The first contains general pronouncements on foodstuffs, in the second he discusses food from seeds and fruits, and in the third from plants and animals.

Qusṭā ibn-Lūqā al-Baʿlabakkī was born about 820. He was a Melchite Christian, and, being well versed in Greek, Syriac and Arabic, he produced numerous translations from the Greek, among which were works of Rufus of Ephesus. Towards the end of his life, following a call from the prince Sanherib, he moved from Baghdad to Armenia, where he died in 912. Qusṭā, who had made a special study of mathematics and philosophy, also composed a number of stimulating medical works. It is obvious that he was particularly interested in physiological and psychological questions. In his book *Kitāb fī ʿIlal ikhtilāf an-nās fī akhlāqi-him wa-siyari-him wa-shahawāti-him wa-khtiyārāti-him* he examined the relations which exist between constitution and character, conduct of life, the emotions and aesthetic perception.[4]

Abū-Bakr Muḥammad ibn-Zakariyyā' ar-Rāzī (latinized as Rhazes) was born in Rayy in 865. After directing the hospitals in Rayy and Baghdad for a while he took to travelling and so reached the court of the Sāmānid prince of Kerman and Khurasan, Abū-Ṣāliḥ Manṣūr ibn-Is'ḥāq, to whom he dedicated the *Kitāb al-Manṣūrī*, which has become one of the great classical works of Arabic medicine. Of its ten parts *Liber Nonus* was especially well known in the West. In this book special pathology is presented with the usual arrangement of illnesses *a capite usque ad calcem*. No less a person than Andreas Vesalius worked further on this ninth part.

The *Kitāb al-Ḥāwī* (*Continens*) is really only a collection of excerpts on pathology and therapy from Greek, Indian and Arabic authors, a vast mass of raw material which ar-Rāzī might have used as the basis of his writings. Occasionally he has also incorporated into this material notes of his own medical observations.[5] Probably he had not intended to publish these excerpts. However, after his death, Ibn-al-ʿAmīd, the vizier of the Buwayhid Rukn-ad-Dawla, got some pupils of ar-Rāzī to publish these notes and scribblings in book form. Thus came into being an enormous work of twenty-three volumes which had a lasting effect on the later medical literature of the Arabs.[6] It was translated into Latin by Faraj ibn-Sālim (in Latin, Faragut) and has long served as a teaching manual in various faculties.

Ar-Rāzī, who died in 923, was just as important as a doctor as he was as philosopher[7] and alchemist. August Müller called him 'the most creative genius of medieval medicine' and Von Grunebaum praised 'the sureness of his diagnosis and the cool precision of his case histories'. That he has made an individual contribution by his description of smallpox and catarrh will be shown later. But one must beware of passing general judgements of this sort as long as a large part of the writings of ar-Rāzī are not accessible in print. It must not be forgotten too, that ar-Rāzī had occasionally recommended treatment by sympathetic magic, so that he could hardly be called a critical rationalist by our standards.

ʿAlī ibn-al-ʿAbbās al-Majūsī came from a Persian Zoroastrian family from al-Ahwāz; he served as a doctor in the service of the Buwayhid prince ʿAḍud-ad-Dawla Fanāʾ Khusrau (*regnabat* 949–82) and died between A.D. 982 and 995. He was *homo unius libri* but his work, the *Kitāb Kāmil aṣ-ṣināʿa aṭ-ṭibbiyya*, also called *al-Kitāb al-Malakī*, is one of the great classical works of Islamic medicine and has been able to maintain its fame alongside the *Canon* of Avicenna right through the Middle Ages and into modern times. It is distinguished by brevity and clarity of presentation but does not escape a certain dryness. It is almost totally free of magical and astrological ideas and represents the schematized Galenism of Arabic medicine in the purest form. I have therefore based my subsequent investigations in the first place on this book.[8]

Abū-l-Qāsim Khalaf ibn-al-ʿAbbās az-Zahrāwī was working as a doctor in Cordova at the time of the caliph ʿAbd-ar-Raḥmān III (*regnabat* 912–61). Of his great work, the *Kitāb at-Taṣrīf*, the thirtieth part, dealing with surgery, has become specially well known. Whereas in other Arabic medical works, surgery was more or less treated as the cinderella, here it is presented very knowledgeably and in great detail. Abū-l-Qāsim has used the sixth book of Paulus of Aegina as his main source but has also added much that is his own. He makes big demands on the surgeons when he says:

> Now this is the reason why there is no skilful operator in our day: the art of medicine is long and it is necessary for its exponent, before he exercises it, to be trained in anatomy as Galen has described it, so that he may be fully

> acquainted with the uses, forms, and temperament of the limbs; also how they are jointed, and how they may be separated; that he should understand fully also the bones, tendons and muscles, their numbers and their attachments; and also the blood vessels, both arteries and veins, with their relations.[9]

As a result, surgery, which up till now had been left to cuppers and barbers, was, thanks to Abū-l-Qāsim, completely integrated into scientific medicine.

The significance of the *Kitāb at-Taṣrīf* does not lie ultimately in the fact that in its Latin version, prepared by Gerard of Cremona, it had a great influence on the surgical works of Roger of Parma, Lanfranchi, Guilielmo Salicetti and Fabrizio d'Acquapendente. Above all, it is often quoted in the *Chirurgia magna* of Guy de Chauliac, completed in 1363, and has thus exercised its influence right into the eighteenth century. There was also a Turkish version of Abū-l-Qāsim's account of surgery which was dedicated to Mehmet, conqueror of Constantinople (*regnabat* 1451–81).

Abū-ʿAlī al-Ḥusayn ibn-ʿAbd-Allāh ibn-Sīnā (in Latin, Avicenna) was born in Afshana near Bukhara in 980 (or a little earlier). His many-sided studies encompassed the Koran, law, logic, metaphysics, mathematics, astronomy and medicine. If one can believe Avicenna's self-conscious autobiography, he was already practising as a doctor at the age of 16. A little later he was called to treat the ruler of Bukhārā, Nūḥ ibn-Manṣūr. In the latter's rich library, he had the opportunity of getting to know the works of many early authors. For political reasons, Avicenna moved between 1002 and 1005 from Bukhārā to Gurgānj; finally, after several moves, he settled in Jurjān. Here he began to write down his main medical work, the *Kitāb al-Qānūn*. Later, in Hamadhān he became vizier of the Buwayhid Shams-ad-Dawla abū-Ṭāhir (*regnabat* 997–1021). In the year 1037 he died in Hamadhān as the result of a colic.[10]

Avicenna's fame as a doctor rests chiefly on the *Qānūn* which he began to write in Jurjān and completed in Hamadhān. Later he wanted to incorporate the experiences he had gained in practice, but the papers on which he had noted them got lost. Even without these, the *Qānūn* is a gigantic work consisting of five books, which in places are further subdivided into subjects, subsidiary subjects, summaries and sections. The first book (*al-kulliyyāt*) is the general part. It deals with physiology, nosology, aetiology, symptomatology and the principles of therapy. In the second book, the simples from the three realms of nature are presented, the strength, effect and use being given exactly. The third book is devoted to special pathology. As usual, diseases are enumerated in the order of where they occur in the body, *a capite ad calcem*. Those illnesses that involve the whole body, for example, fevers, ulcers, fractures and poisonings, are dealt with in the fourth book. Finally, the fifth book is the dispensary, the apothecary's book, in which the mixing of drugs is taught.

The *Qānūn* has won the highest esteem both in the East and in the West. This is shown by the mass of manuscripts preserved even to this day, and by the great number of commentaries, supercommentaries, epitomes, glosses, imitations and translations. About 100 years after Avicenna's death, Gerard of Cremona in Toledo translated the *Qānūn* into Latin. Andrea Alpago (d. 1522), the great doctor and orientalist, who worked for many years in Damascus, the seat of the Venetian consulate, improved this translation.[11] The Latin *Canon* was then printed thirty-six times in the fifteenth and sixteenth centuries. Yet, however great the influence of this book may have been, its significance really lies only in the systematization and comprehensive presentation of the medical science of the time. No personal experiences of the author and no new ideas are to be found in it. The Ferranese doctor Giovanni Manardi (d. 1536) wrote: 'Constat Auicennam totum fere suum de medicina librum ex aliis medicis, tum Graecis, tum barbaris, transcripsisse.' In the future the task will be to uncover the sources of the great compilation–a difficult task, because Avicenna seldom mentions his sources by name, and because he does not quote the texts verbatim but freely changes and adapts them.

Abū-Marwān ʿAbd-al-Malik ibn-Zuhr (in Latin Avenzoar) was born in Seville in 1091 or 1094. At first he served the Almoravids and dedicated his first work, the *Kitāb al-Iqtiṣād*, to Ibrāhīm ibn-Yūsuf ibn-Tāshufīn, whom he extolled as patron of the sciences, as bibliophile, and as one well versed in the works of Galen. Arrested by ʿAlī ibn-Yūsuf ibn-Tāshufīn,

Ibn-Zuhr languished for roughly ten years in prison in Marrakesh. After the seizure of power by the Almohads, he became vizier and personal physician to ʿAbd-al-Mu'min (*regnabat* 1130–63), and was able to spend the last fifteen years of his life in Spain again. Here he wrote the *Kitāb at-Taysīr*, his main work. Soon after its completion Ibn-Zuhr died in Seville in 1161–2. The *Taysīr* is a book on pathology, with a collection of prescriptions. It contains the 'Particularia' of medicine, to complement which Averroes may be said to have written his '*Generalia*'. The reputation which Avenzoar enjoyed in Europe is founded on the *Taysīr*, which was translated into Hebrew and Latin. The work was printed eight times in Latin between 1490 and 1554.

Abū-l-Walīd Muḥammad ibn-Aḥmad ibn-Rushd (in Latin Averroes) was born in Cordova in 1126. Basically a jurist, he busied himself chiefly with philosophy and was the most important interpreter of Aristotle in the Islamic Middle Ages. He was employed as a state official in Cordova and Marrakesh, and died in the year 1198.[12] His main medical work is the *Kitāb al-Kulliyyāt*, which became known in a Latin translation under the title '*Colliget*'. As already stated, these '*Generalia*' were regarded as a counterpart of the '*Particularia*' of Avenzoar. The seven parts of the work deal with anatomy, dietetics, pathology, symptomatology, nourishment, materia medica, hygiene and therapeutics. By this division of the subject Averroes was consciously following a short article by al-Fārābī, in which the latter demands that the doctor should master these seven areas.[13] At the same time Averroes makes clear that the 'Generalia' of medicine fall within the competence of the philosopher, and thus differences between Galen and Aristotle in physiological questions are to be decided in favour of the latter.

The great Jewish philosopher Abū-ʿImrān Mūsā ibn-ʿUbayd-Allāh ibn-Maymūn (in Latin Maimonides) was born in Cordova on 30 March 1135. When the Almohads forced him to leave his home, he settled in Egypt and served Saladin's son al-Malik al-Afḍal Nūr-ad-Dīn ʿAlī as personal physician. Maimonides died in 1204.[14] The most famous of his works is the *Aphorisms*, the *Kitāb al-Fuṣūl*,[15] a collection of 1500 quotations from Galen's writings, divided according to theme into twenty-five chapters. Occasionally Maimonides quotes Arab authors also, for example, Muḥammad ibn-Aḥmad at-Tamīmī, Abū-Marwān ibn-Zuhr, ibn-at-Tilmīdh and others. In the twenty-fifth chapter Maimonides critically dissects those passages in Galen's works which seemed to him problematical. Maimonides also wrote two *Regimina sanitatis*[16] for his master afflicted by melancholy, and worked a number of Galen's writings into the form of a compendium. He also wrote about poisons and collected synonyms of drugs.

Muwaffaq-ad-Dīn ʿAbd-al-Laṭīf ibn-Yūsuf al-Baghdādī was born in Baghdad in 1162. After studying philology, theology, philosophy and alchemy, he travelled to Damascus, Cairo and other cities. Later he turned more to the ancient authors, especially to Aristotle and Alexander of Aphrodisias. From 1207 he taught medicine in Damascus. After undertaking journeys in Anatolia and making the pilgrimage to Mecca, he died in Baghdad in 1231. 'Abd-al-Laṭīf's autobiography reveals that its author was a man of great originality of character, and a scholar of independent thought who strove passionately for what was known to be right. At the same time he was a man who made fierce attacks on colleagues and on his erstwhile idols, Avicenna and alchemy. We will find this confirmed later when we discuss his discovery of the unity of the lower maxilla and his book on diabetes.[17]

Another teacher of medicine in Damascus was ʿAlā'-ad-Dīn ʿAlī ibn-Abī-l-Ḥazm al-Qurashī, called Ibn-an-Nafīs, who died in 1288. As a theological writer he came out with the rather dry treatise *Fāḍil ibn-Nāṭiq*.[18] In addition to commentaries on several Hippocratic writings Ibn-an-Nafīs wrote an epitome of the *Canon* of Avicenna, a practical manual, extremely widely known and very popular, and later frequently commented on. Further he produced a large commentary on the *Canon*, in which he developed his theory of pulmonary circulation, which we shall go into later (p. 68f.).

Diyā'-ad-Dīn ʿAbd-Allāh ibn-Aḥmad ibn-al-Bayṭar was born in Malaga towards the end of the twelfth century. About 1220 he travelled to the East, and after journeyings in North Africa, Asia Minor and Syria, settled in Egypt, where the sultan al-Kāmil Muḥammad (*regnabat* 1218–38) bestowed on him the title of 'chief of botanists'. He died in Damascus in 1248. Ibn-al-Bayṭar wrote several works on materia medica, of which the *Kitāb al-Jāmi' li-mufradāt al-adwiya wa-l-aghdhiya*, a gigantic work about remedies and food, is especially well known. It is only a collection of excerpts, however, a compilation from more than two hundred different sources. In it, for example, the complete text of Dioscurides has been taken over.

The names mentioned here are only a small selection from the many dozens of famous doctors or prolific medical writers which the Islamic middle ages produced. Some further names will be mentioned in the following chapters in connection with specific pathological themes about which these doctors wrote. In the circumstances new discoveries or new systematic thinking could scarcely be expected from the medieval doctors. In essence the ancient teachings were only reproduced, and most books and treatises are compilations whose content became ever shallower as time went on.

Naturally one must not judge the position of medicine in Islamic countries solely on the basis of the writings of the doctors. Doctors in any case were to be found only in the large cities, and most of the well-known names were either personal physicians to the sultans or else professors, and had reached a high level of culture. The urban poor and the rural population were practically deprived of all medical help, and in these areas when anyone offered aid to a sick person he was either a quack or a very ignorant doctor. The situation throughout the Middle Ages was probably similar to that which obtained in Aleppo in the eighteenth century, and about which we possess an excellent and detailed account by Alexander Russell (d. 1768), physician to the British factory in Aleppo for twenty years.[19] According to Russell medicine was not so much in the hands of the Turks as in those of the Christians and Jews. In order to practise, it was necessary to have a licence from the Hakim Bashi, but this could be gained for a financial consideration. The student received no systematic training either at the bedside or through study. The medicines were prepared by the doctors themselves. Diagnosis by feeling the pulse played a large role; surgery was extremely neglected. 'Their [i.e. the physicians'] knowledge of anatomy is acquired by reading, not from dissection, and both anatomy and physiology remain precisely in the state in which they were transmitted by Galen' (p. 132).

The decline of Arabic medicine is also shown by the fact that important personages often had no doctor at their disposal. In 1471 the Portuguese king Alfonso v had taken Arzila, a small coastal town between Tangier and Larache, and the garrison stationed there was always provided with one or two military surgeons. When Mūlāy Ibrāhīm, the vizier of the sultan Aḥmad ibn-Muḥammad al-Waṭṭāsī, fell ill in 1530 at Shauen, he called the doctor Duarte Rodrigues from Arzila; and in 1532 when his sister Lalla ʿĀ'isha, the wife of the sultan, fell ill, he again asked the Portuguese to make a visit.[20] It should not of course be assumed that at that time European medicine was theoretically superior to Arabic medicine. The Arabic tradition still dominated medicine in Europe, as is seen from the numerous editions of Avicenna produced in the fifteenth and sixteenth centuries. What the above incident proves is that the Sultan of Morocco at that time had no comparable doctor in his service; and this is so far typical and shows the change which was occurring in the sciences of the East and the West.

The influence of Europe on Islamic medicine makes itself emphatically felt in the seventeenth century, when Ṣāliḥ ibn-Naṣr-Allāh ibn-Sallūm, physician to the Ottoman sultan Mehmet iv, wrote his *Kitāb Ghāyat al-itqān fī tadbīr badan al-insān*. In this work we find not only the description of 'new' illnesses, which were unknown in classical times, for example, chlorosis, syphilis, scurvy and Polish plait (plica polonica), but an altogether new system, namely the 'chemical medicine of Paracelsus'. Ibn-Sallūm, who was born in Aleppo and had presumably had the opportunity to learn Latin from European doctors, here bases himself on the *Paramirum* of Paracelsus, though he may have known this only indirectly through the writings of Paracelsus's pupil Oswald Crollius. Ibn-Sallūm here develops pathology, not from Galen's theory of humours, but from the three basic substances, salt, quicksilver and sulphur, and teaches a therapy using the philosopher's stone, the universal remedy.

When a century later in 1767 the plague was raging in Istanbul, against which traditional Islamic medicine could do nothing, the sultan Muṣṭafā iii, hoping for effective relief, had Turkish translations made of Herman Boerhaave's *Institutiones medicinae* (first published at Leiden in 1707) and *Aphorismi de cognoscendis et curandis morbis* (Leiden 1709). The work was carried out by the court physician Ṣubḥī-Zāde ʿAbd-al-ʿAzīz, who enlisted the help of the Imperial Austrian interpreter Thomas von Herbert, and was completed in 1768. It was not a literal translation, but rather an adaptation, because Ṣubḥī-Zāde was trying by means of explanations and additions to harmonize this modern medicine with the traditional views.[21] These translations of Boerhaave, however, hardly received a wide circulation, and so remained without influence. It became clear, however, from the translations of Paracelsus and Boerhaave that new advances in medicine need no longer be expected from the Orient. It was only in the nineteenth century, however, that the great change-over took place.

Antoine-Barthélemy Clot, born in Grenoble in 1793, did most to introduce scientific medicine into Egypt. In 1820 he became doctor of Medicine at Montpellier and in 1823 doctor of surgery. In 1825 he was appointed surgeon-in-chief to the Egyptian army by Muḥammad ʿAlī. By 1828 he had founded a medical school at Abū-Zaʿbal near Cairo, which was later enlarged to include pharmaceutical and veterinary sections and a midwifery ward; it was transferred to Cairo in 1837. Other French professors taught there as well as Italians and Germans. Clot carried out important surgical operations, which he wrote up in numerous papers, but he had difficulty in obtaining permission to dissect corpses. On the occasion of the great plague of 1835 he adopted the opinion of the anticontagionists and spurned the quarantine regulations.[22]

In Iran instruction in modern scientific subjects began only in 1850 with the founding of the Dār al-funūn in Teheran, a medical and military school which was to train officers and doctors, the latter also for civilian duty. Its founder was the grand vizier Mīrzā Taqī Khān, who on diplomatic journeys to Europe recognized the need for this step. The teachers at the Dār al-funūn were Austrians and Italians, and the language of instruction was French.[23]

Since then, however, and up to the present day the situation in Islamic countries is characterized by the coexistence of traditional Arabic medicine and modern European medicine. When cholera raged in Egypt in the summer of 1883, and the French and German mission under Louis Pasteur and Robert Koch came to Egypt to study the epidemic, the leading doctors in Cairo and Alexandria were almost entirely European.[24] At the same time, however, Arabic medicine was fully asserting its validity. The Bulaq editions of the great works of Ibn-al-Bayṭār (1874), Avicenna and al-Majūsī (both 1877) were not occasioned by an interest in the history of medicine, but by the fact that they contained a living, practical medicine.

In India right down to the present day Unānī medicine, that is, Greek medicine transmitted through Arabic and Persian sources, is practised alongside ayurvedic and modern European medicine. Here the tradition, especially that nurtured by the Bahmanids in the Deccan from the fourteenth to the sixteenth century and by the Mogul emperors in Hindustan (1525–1857), was never broken off. The main text-book of this Unānī medicine is as always the *Canon* of Avicenna, together with the commentaries and elaborations like the *Mūjiz* of Ibn-an-Nafīs and the *Qānūnja* of Maḥmūd ibn-ʿUmar al-Jaghmīnī (d. after 1221); these were highly valued and published in lithographed editions in the nineteenth century. This medical tradition is indeed attacked and contested from within its own ranks. In 1878 Ḥakīm Afḍal ʿAlī from Fyzabad wrote a book with the title *Jāmiʿash-shifāʾiyya* in which he explained that Greek medicine rested on false assumptions. Even after that, however, Masīḥ-al-Mulk Ḥakīm Muḥammad Ajmal Khān was able, with the support of the Indian government, to found the Ayurvedi and the Unānī Ṭibbī College in Delhi.[25]

The influence of Arabic medicine on the West

In a survey of the history of Arabic medicine, however cursory, the role played by this medicine in the Latin Middle Ages must not go unmentioned. We have already remarked from time to time that a number of writings by Ḥunayn ibn-Is'ḥāq, ar-Rāzī, az-Zahrāwī and Ibn-Sīnā had been translated into Latin. How did this meeting of Arabic and Western medicine come about?

Up to the tenth century the writings of ancient authors had for the most part fallen into oblivion in the West, and only in a few places were the early medieval Latin translations of some writings of Galen still in existence. For the rest men relied on what was said in general compilations like the *Etymologiae* of

Isidore of Seville on the subject of human anatomy. Moreover the scientific standards of the old medical school at Salerno had sunk to a low level.

About the middle of the eleventh century, however, this was radically altered by the appearance of Constantinus Africanus. Of his life little is known. What is reported generally bears legendary traits and can hardly be considered as historically reliable. Constantinus must have been born at the beginning of the eleventh century in Tunis. When he was forty, he is said to have come to Italy, perhaps as a merchant. After seeing the pitiful state of medicine there, he went back to Tunis to study medicine for three years and then finally settled in Italy. He was converted to Christianity and became a monk in the Benedictine monastery of Monte Cassino where he spent the rest of his life translating the Arabic books he had brought with him. He died at Monte Cassino in 1087.

Constantinus translated into Latin the most important of the Arabic medical works which had appeared up to the middle of the eleventh century. They were then for the most part circulated under his own name, as if he, not an Arab, was the author. The *Liber Constantini de melancholia* is none other than the *Maqāla fī l-Mālankhūliyā* of Is'ḥāq ibn-'Imrān, the *Liber de oblivione* is the *Risāla fī n-Nisyān wa-'ilāji-hī* of Ibn-al-Jazzār. Constantinus also translated under the title *Viaticum peregrinantis* another work by Ibn-al-Jazzār, the *Kitāb Zād al-musāfir*, a sketch of general medicine. The *Kitāb al-Malakī* of al-Majūsī became the *Liber Pantegni*. In addition there were several writings by Is'ḥāq ibn-Sulaymān al-Isrā'īlī (Isaac Judaeus). Constantinus's translations are difficult to understand because they are too wordy and because he retains Arabic technical terms. Despite this his influence was felt to be so significant that Petrus Diaconus could call him 'orientis et occidentis magister, novusque effulgens Hippocrates'. Even if one does not share this emphatic contemporary judgement, yet it is certain that the school of Salerno was revived by Constantinus, and that beyond this European medicine was quite definitely influenced and fertilized through him.

In 1085 Toledo was won back by the Christians, but many Arabs and Arabic-speaking Jews remained under Christian rule. In 1125 Raymond of Sauvetât became archbishop of

Toledo. He realized that Toledo provided an opportunity for the translation of the Arabic scientific works into Latin, and the town soon became the centre where Arabic learning was passed on to the West. Domenicus Gundissalinus (Domingo Gonzalez) and Joannes Hispalensis were leading translators in the spheres of Arabic philosophy and the exact sciences. They were joined in 1150 by Gerard, who was born in Cremona in Lombardy in 1114 but now came to Toledo to study Arabic texts, especially the *Almagest* of Ptolemy. Gerard translated not only the *Almagest*, but also the great medical compendia of ar-Rāzī, az-Zahrāwī and Ibn-Sīnā. About a hundred works are ascribed to him, but these cannot possibly all stem from him. What happened to Gerard's name is no different from what happened to Ḥunayn's; to these famous translators were ascribed all those works whose translator was unknown.

A further name must be mentioned: Stephen of Pisa. He studied in Salerno, and after a short stay in Sicily went to Antioch in Syria in 1127, and there he made a new translation of the *Kitāb al-Malakī* by al-Majūsī. This version, which is better known than that of Constantinus, bears the title *Liber regius*.[26]

These translations of the eleventh and twelfth centuries laid the foundations of the 'Arabism' in the medicine of the West, that trend which was dominant for centuries, and was reversed only in modern times and after long arguments. For long the rule held that he who would be a good doctor must be a good Avicennist.[27]

FOUR

PHYSIOLOGY AND ANATOMY

In this chapter the basic physiological, anatomical and pathological conceptions of the Arabs will be described. Knowledge of these is the prerequisite for an understanding of Arabic medical literature and of the thinking of Islamic doctors. The physiological and pathological views change from author to author in greater or lesser degree. One cannot therefore speak of the 'physiology of the Arabs' because by so doing, one would be presenting an average view which would be unhistorical. Rather one must concentrate on one author whose teachings in a particular case can be compared or contrasted with those of another.

In order to sketch the basic characteristics, I have chosen the *Kitāb al-Malakī* of ʿAlī ibn-al-ʿAbbās al-Majūsī. Al-Majūsī's express aim[1] was to write a book which embraces everything that the student of medicine needs until he is master of his art. By this work, which was not to be prolix, but was with all brevity to present clearly everything that concerns health and illness, the student should become independent of all other medical books. This programme is a massive literary Topos. But al-Majūsī's book–one of the largest works of Arabic medical literature–indeed excels itself in its lucidity and its noteworthy clarity of presentation. It was highly valued in the Middle Ages, and was translated twice into Latin; and even today more than a hundred Arabic manuscripts of it are preserved. Al-Majūsī's system marks the end of the development of the medical thought of the ancients. The author is an out-and-out Galenist, though he does not link up directly with individual writings of Galen but is in the tradition of the late Alexandrian school with its synopsis of Galen, a tradition which also determined the *Kitāb al-Mudkhal* of Ḥunayn ibn-

Is'ḥāq. This can be shown in what follows in some particular points.

The elements

The philosophers mean by an element the simplest part of a composite body and that with the smallest measurement.[2] A thing is 'simple' when its substance (*jawhar*) is homogeneous and its parts are similar. This is really (*bi-l-ḥaqīqa*) so in the case of fire, air, water and earth. But stones and minerals also appear 'simple' to the senses. However, these are only made up of fire, air, etc., which ought to be called the 'primary' elements (*al-ustuquṣṣāt al-uwal*) in contrast to the 'secondary' and 'tertiary' elements (*ath-thawānī*, *ath-thawālith*). One can also say that there are 'near and special' (*qarība*, *khāṣṣa*) elements, 'distant and general' (*ba'īda*, *'āmma*) elements, and elements 'lying in the middle'.

An example will help to explain this: In a warm-blooded animal, the 'near elements' are the homoeomeral organs because all 'instrumental' organs of the body are composed of these. The 'middle elements' are the four humours because the homoeomeral organs are composed of these. The 'distant elements' are the primary general elements, namely, fire, air, water and earth. Out of their mixing the plants arise, these are used for the food of animals, from the food are produced the humours, from the humours are produced the homoeomeral organs, from the homoeomeral organs are produced the instrumental organs, and of these the whole body is composed. However, with the senses we cannot perceive the four elements in their pure state but we can grasp them only with the reason, for the fire that we see is always sullied with dust and smoke, the water that we find, always has earthy components. This means that the elements as such nowhere appear. They are abstract, ideal quantities which underlie the concrete.

The elements (*ustuquṣṣāt*) can be defined as the hot, the cold, the wet and the dry; but by these are not meant the qualities themselves but the substances (*jawāhir*) in which those qualities are expressed in the highest degree. The hot substance in the highest degree is fire, the cold susbtance in the highest degree water, the moist substance in the highest degree air, and the dry substance in the highest degree earth. Actually these elements or qualities, because of their propinquity, occur only in mixed forms; fire gains a dry quality, air a hot, water a wet, and earth a cold. This means that the 'power' of fire is hot-dry, that of air hot-wet, of water cold-wet and of earth cold-dry.

The temperament

Everything that exists in the world of growth and decay has thus arisen out of the four elements, when they are mixed with one another in different amounts and unequal proportions. This relationship of mixing in organic bodies is called 'temperament' (*krāsis*, *mizāj*).[3] A body in which the elements are equally present is called 'balanced' or 'even' (*muʿtadil*); if its elements are present in unequal proportions, it is said to be 'unbalanced' (*khārij ʿan al-iʿtidāl*). If the fiery element is dominant, the temperament is called hot; if the watery element is dominant the temperament is said to be cold. If the element of air is dominant together with the fiery element, the temperament is designated 'hot-wet', and so on. There are thus nine different temperaments, one that is balanced, and eight out of balance. Of the latter four are simple and four composite.

In addition every temperament may have a stronger or a weaker stamp, so that there is an endless number of gradations, which comes to expression in the endless differences between individuals. Added to these we have external factors which can influence temperament, namely, the land or clime in which a person is born and brought up, his age, his sex and his habit; this last according to Hippocrates is a second nature. In all kinds of animals, for example, the male is always hotter and drier than the female. The habit of eating much can make an originally thin body fat. Occupational activity leads the glassmaker to become hot and dry, the bath attendant hot and wet, fishermen and sailors cold and wet.

The four humours (al-akhlāṭ)

The humours were designated above as the 'middle' or 'secondary' elements. All organs of men and of animals possessing blood are created from the four humours, namely, blood, phlegm, yellow bile and black bile.[4] These humours are called 'daughters of the elements' (*banāt al-arkān*), because relationships exist between the humours and the elements. Fire corresponds to yellow bile, which is hot and dry; air corresponds to blood which is hot and wet; water corresponds to phlegm which is cold and wet, and earth corresponds to black bile which is cold and dry: if these four humours form a balanced mixture, then there is health. If the balance is quantitatively or qualitatively disturbed, then illness ensues.

Blood is produced in the liver from the juice of the digested food. The blood in the arteries is of fine consistency, it is pure red with sometimes a tendency to reddish-yellow. The blood in the veins holds the balance between fine and coarse; it is dark red, has a sweet taste and quickly coagulates when it comes out. This blood is produced when the heat of the liver is lessened. If there is too great a degree of heat and dryness in the liver, the blood becomes muddy and coarse; if there is too much wet and cold, the blood becomes thin and watery. If the liver is too cold, the colour of the blood tends to be white. The pure red, on the other hand, comes from too much yellow bile being mixed with the blood.

Natural phlegm is cold and wet. Phlegm remains naturally in the veins where it digests, matures, and is prepared for the nourishing of the organs. There are four kinds of unnatural phlegm; the acid is very cold and dry, the salty is very hot and dry, the sweet is very hot and wet, and that which resembles molten glass is very cold, wet and coarse and cannot change into blood.

Natural yellow bile is fine (*laṭīf*) and its colour pure red. The finest, sharpest and purest-coloured type is drawn from the gall-bladder. This sends part of the yellow bile into the bowels in order to wash away the phlegm from them, another part goes to the stomach to help it digest food. The yellow bile which is least sharp and pure-coloured flows with the blood through the whole body. It is supposed to refine and thin the blood in order that it can penetrate the narrow vessels so that the organs can be nourished by the blood. There are four types of unnatural yellow bile; the first is yellow-coloured; it is produced by the mixing of pure red bile with the watery moisture.

The second type resembles egg-yolk; it is produced by the mixing of pure red bile with the coarse phlegm-like moisture. Both these types arise in the liver. The third type has the colour of leeks; it arises chiefly in the stomach through the enjoyment of vegetables. The fourth type has the colour of verdigris. This is a bad type; its quality corresponds to the poison of poisonous animals; it arises in the stomach as the result of 'burning'.[5]

The natural type of black bile is called 'the black humour' (*melas khymos*, *al-khilṭ as-sawdāwī*). It arises chiefly as the result of a cool dry diet and is to the blood what yeast is to wine. The spleen attracts the coarsest parts of this humour and nourishes itself with the best of it. It directs the rest to the mouth of the stomach (that is, the upper end of the stomach, Greek: *kardia*) so as to stimulate the appetite. The less coarse components of the black humour reach the whole body with the blood in the veins so as to nourish those organs that need coarse, cold food, for example, the bones and cartilage. The unnatural type of this humour is called 'black bile' in the narrower sense (*melaina kholē*, *al-mirra as-sawdā'*).[6] It arises out of the burning of the 'black humour' and is hot and sharp; its taste is acid. A further type arises from the burning of 'yellow bile'. This type is hotter and sharper than the former; it is dark black and gleams like pitch. It nourishes malignant diseases like cancer, elephantiasis (*judhām*), malignant tumours etc. The cause of its origin is a hot, dry diet. Finally, there are varieties of black bile which are pale grey, or the colour of the aubergine or violet.

Now it must be noted that there are humours that can change into others and some which cannot.[7] Phlegm can turn into blood when the 'innate heat' (*to emphyton thermon*, *al-ḥarāra al-gharīziyya*) works on it and allows it to mature. Blood turns into yellow bile if strong heat makes it thin; but blood cannot turn into phlegm. Yellow bile often becomes black bile if strong heat 'burns' it; but yellow bile cannot become blood or phlegm. Black bile can become neither blood nor phlegm, nor yellow bile. These four humours therefore represent four different degrees of maturation or 'cooking'. This 'cooking' process cannot be undone because cooked food cannot become raw again.

It must also be noted that every humour, when it predominates in a whole body, or quantitatively or qualitatively in an organ, calls forth an illness corresponding to the humour. The absence too of a humour leads to a specific illness. If there is a superfluity of a humour present, so that it fills the organs, it suffocates the innate heat and so leads to death.

The faculties

The whole physiological process is governed and directed by the interplay of different faculties.[8] There are three basic faculties: 1) the natural faculties (*al-quwā aṭ-ṭabīʿiyya*) are the effects of nature which manifest themselves in conception, growth and nourishment; 2) the animal faculties (*al-quwā al-ḥayawāniyya*) ensure life; they manifest themselves in the systole and diastole of the heart and arteries; 3) the psychical faculties determine the reason, the power of discernment, emotion and voluntary movement. The natural faculties also belong to animals and plants, the animal faculties belong to both rational and irrational animals, but man alone possesses psychical faculties.

1. The seat of the natural faculties is the liver. From it they are carried along the veins to the organs, which in this way receive these faculties. The procreative faculty produces the foetus from the male sperm and the menstrual blood. It is effective from the moment of conception until the embryo is fully grown. It is supported by two other faculties, namely, by the first transforming faculty (*al-quwwa al-mughayyira al-ūlā*), which transforms the substance of the sperm and the menstrual blood into the substance of the foetal organs, and the form-giving faculty which gives the organs and limbs the forms they will assume. The faculty of growth allows the organs and limbs of the foetus to grow quantitatively. It is at work from the beginning of foetal development until the end of adolescence. It supports the procreative faculty and is in turn supported by the nourishing faculty. The nourishing faculty replaces the used-up materials in the organs without increasing the organs quantitatively. It is active from the beginning of foetal development until death. It serves, as mentioned, the growth faculty but is itself supported by four

other 'natural faculties'. These are: a) the attractive faculty (*al-quwwa al-jādhiba*), b) the retentive faculty (*al-quwwa al-māsika*), c) the second transforming faculty (*al-quwwa al-mughayyira ath-thāniya*) and d) the excretory faculty (*al-quwwa ad-dāfiʿa*).

The attractive faculty procures for the organs nourishment peculiar to them and suited to them. The brain, for example, draws cold and wet blood, the bones draw cold and dry blood, the gall-bladder attracts the gall-component of the blood, the kidneys attract the watery waste matter. These drawing faculties work physically through a vacuum, through heat (as in the case of the flame which draws the oil through the wick) or by a natural property (as with magnets). The retentive faculty retains a suitable substance in an organ until it is digested or transformed; it works above all through cold and dryness. The second transforming faculty is also called the digestive faculty (*al-quwwa al-hāḍima*). It turns the nourishment suitable for an organ into the substance of this organ and works by means of heat and moisture.[9] The excretory faculty finally removes from an organ the waste matter in those materials which the attractive faculty has produced. It works with the help of heat and dryness.

2. Life is maintained by the animal faculties.[10] They are located in the heart, and they reach the organs by the arteries and give them life. Some of these faculties are active, for example, the faculty which effects the systole and diastole of the heart and arteries, others are passive, for example, the faculties which produce anger and pride. Anger arises if one of the agents coming from without sets the 'innate heat' in motion. Anger is namely the surging up of the heart's blood and the sudden emergence of the innate heat on the surface of the body when a thirst for revenge has to be satisfied.

3. The seat of the psychical faculties is the brain.[11] There are three types: a) faculties in which the brain operates autonomously, by which it rules (*to hēgemonikon*, *al-mudabbir*), as well as faculties which the brain uses by means of the nerves, b) the perceptions of the senses, c) voluntary movement. The dominant faculties are reason and thought (*adh-dhihn wa-l-fikr*). They can be further subdivided into imagination (*takhayyul*), thought (*fikr*), and memory (*dhikr*), that is, into abilities, each

of which is located in definite ventricles of the brain. The perceptive faculties (*al-quwā al-ḥassāsa*) are those faculties that determine the sensations. The faculties which cause voluntary movement (*al-ḥaraka al-irādiyya*), operate through the fact that something of the substance of the 'psychical pneuma' (*ar-rūḥ an-nafsānī*), which is located in the ventricles of the brain, presses through the nerves to the limbs.

The pneumata

The 'faculties' have their correlation in the 'pneumata'. The pneuma, which played a central role not only in medical physiology but also in philosophical psychology from the beginnings until well into the Christian world view, is the link between the material and spiritual nature of man. It is a 'mechanical-dynamic principle' which, in conjunction with the 'innate heat', organizes or breaks down the material.[12] The condition of the body and the carrying through of its functions depend on the pneumata. They, too, are of three types: 1) the natural pneuma (*ar-rūḥ aṭ-ṭabīʿī*), 2) the animal pneuma (*ar-rūḥ al-ḥayawānī*) and 3) the psychical pneuma (*ar-rūḥ an-nafsānī*).

1. The natural pneuma originates in the liver, is taken through the veins to the organs and there supports the function of the 'natural faculties'. This pneuma originates in the best, purest and finest blood in the liver, not mixed with any other humour or waste matter.

2. The animal pneuma originates in the heart; it reaches the organs through the arteries and there maintains the 'animal faculties'. This pneuma originates in a mixture of fine, pure vapour of the blood and the inhaled air.

3. The psychical pneuma has its seat in the ventricles of the brain, reaches the organs through the nerves and maintains the 'psychical faculties'. This pneuma arises from the animal pneuma situated in the heart in that this rises up from the heart to the brain through the two arteries called carotid (*ʿirqā s-subāt*). These then divide up into the net-like web (the *rete mirabile*, *diktyoeides plegma*, *nasīja shabīha bi-sh-shabaka*), in which the animal pneuma grows up into the psychical pneuma. This pneuma, situated in the posterior ventricle of the brain,

influences movement and memory; the one in the front ventricle influences sense perception, conception and fantasy; that in the middle ventricle influences thinking.

Recapitulation

If one surveys this whole physiological system, one is struck by the stark schematism that is followed relentlessly. This schematism makes it necessary to a certain extent to depart from Galen's teaching. In Galen's works, the *pneuma physikon* plays no role;[13] here, however, it is taken over from Plato or Aristotle to produce a trichotomy. Corresponding to the three psychical powers, three ventricles in the brain are assumed, whereas Galen speaks of four ventricles, two lateral, one middle, and one posterior, which leads to the spinal cord.[14] It is noteworthy that the 'faculties' are thought of in a certain sense as material, because they have their origin in certain cardinal organs and can be further conveyed through the veins or arteries. The veins especially have to perform a massive task in this system; they convey blood, phlegm, yellow bile, the 'black humour', the 'natural faculties' and the 'natural pneuma'.

Terminologically the presentation is not fully developed, and this rather hinders conceptual clarity. The process of forming scientific technical terms has come neither here nor later, to any final conclusion. The *pneuma zōtikon*, 'the vital pneuma' has become in Arabic, as a result of wrong translation, '*rūḥ ḥayawānī*', 'animal pneuma'. For 'element', *ustuquṣṣ* and *rukn* are used interchangeably and by 'element' are indicated not only the smallest substances but also the humours and the homoeomeral organs, so that one must distinguish between 'primary', 'secondary' and 'tertiary' elements. Equivocal is also the concept *ṭabīʿī*, 'natural', which at one time is used in the sense of 'healthy, normally functioning' (as in the case of the humours), and then again in the sense of 'physical' (as in the case of the faculties and pneumata). However, these weaknesses could not damage the system. Since it had been brought into agreement with fundamental philosophical teaching, it appeared evident. By its strong structure and the possibilities of combining individual parts, it was so capable of variety that by it all physiological and pathological appearances could be fully explained. This constituted its strength and ensured its value down to the present day.

The movement of the blood

These basic, general physiological doctrines form the foundation for special physiology, that is, the doctrines about the digestion, the blood-movement, sense perception, and so on. Of these, only the doctrine of the movement of the blood will be discussed in detail. To this, an Islamic doctor, Ibn-an-Nafīs, has contributed an original essay. But first we shall deal with the system of the movement of the blood in the liver, as presented by al-Majūsī.[15]

The food 'cooked' and prepared in the stomach by the 'first digestion' (*al-haḍm al-awwal*) passes through the pylorus (*ho pylōros*, *al-bawwāb*) into the duodenum (*al-mi'ā dhū l-ithnay 'ashara iṣba'an*) and from there into the small intestine (*al-mi'ā ad-daqīq*). There the veins absorb the chyle (*'uṣārat al-ghidhā'*) and transport it through the portal vein (*hē epi pylais phleps*, *al-'irq al-ma'rūf bi-l-bāb*) into the liver, where the 'transforming faculty' changes it into the substance of blood. The blood is then brought through the great vena cava (*al-'irq al-'aẓīm al-ma'rūf bi-l-ajwaf*) to the organs of the body.

Thus the veins (*al-'urūq ghayr aḍ-ḍawārib*) have their point of exit in the liver.[16] They are of looser, softer substance and only possess one wall. They transport the nourishment from the intestines to the liver, and the blood from the liver to the organs so that these can feed themselves with it. The arteries (*al-'urūq aḍ-ḍawārib* or *ash-sharāyīn*) have a double partition. The fibres of the inner layer are striped obliquely and are hard and coarse, the fibres of the outer layer, on the other hand, are horizontally striped and soft. This must be so because the horizontally striped fibres operate the movement of the diastole by means of which the air (*al-hawā'*) from the heart is sucked into it. The oblique striped fibres of the inner layer operate the movement of the systole (*inqibāḍ*) whereby the smoke-like excess (*al-faḍl ad-dukhānī*) is pushed out.

The heart, whose flesh is firm, is made up of different layers of fibres and it likewise has its basis in the diastolic and systolic movements.[17] The heart is surrounded on all sides by the lungs, it has a conical shape, its point inclines to the left because the 'animal spirit' has its seat on this side of the heart; from there too, the arteries radiate outwards and thus one can feel the pulse beat on the left side. The heart has a right and a left ventricle which are separated by a partition. In this partition there is a passage (*manfadh*) which many people (Aristotle is meant) call a 'third ventricle', but this is incorrect.

The right ventricle has two openings. The vena cava which brings the blood from the liver, enters by one of these. This opening is provided with three small membranes, which after the entry of the blood lie on top of one another like a valve, preventing the return of the blood into the vena cava. From the second opening there emerges the vein which has the structure of an artery and which is therefore called 'the arterial vein' (*al-ʿirq ash-shiryānī*).

From the left ventricle of the heart (*at-tajwīf al-aysar*) two arteries go out. The smaller has only a single soft loose wall and is therefore called 'the venous artery' (*ash-shiryān al-ʿirqī*). It transports a great part of the blood and pneuma into the lungs so that these can nourish themselves. There it divides into many branches and takes in air. It transports the air from the lungs to the heart in the opposite direction. The second and larger artery is known as the 'aorta' (*al-awurṭā* or *al-ʿirq al-abhar*) and is divided into two parts of which one goes upwards, the other downwards. The latter is stronger than the ascending one because it has to look after more organs. From the aorta all further arteries of the body branch off.

The two ventricles pulsate in unison, but the left one does so more strongly because it contains a greater amount of blood, animal spirit and innate heat. The right ventricle contains only blood, and only in a small amount. The passage that leads from the right to the left ventricle gradually tapers off in the direction of the left ventricle, so that only the finest constituents of the blood which has come from the liver pass through. The function of the heart consists finally in the fact that it is the storehouse and source of the 'innate heat' (*to emphyton thermon, al-ḥarāra al-gharīziyya*) by which life is maintained.

To understand al-Majūsī's account we must free ourselves completely from what is taught today. His statements about

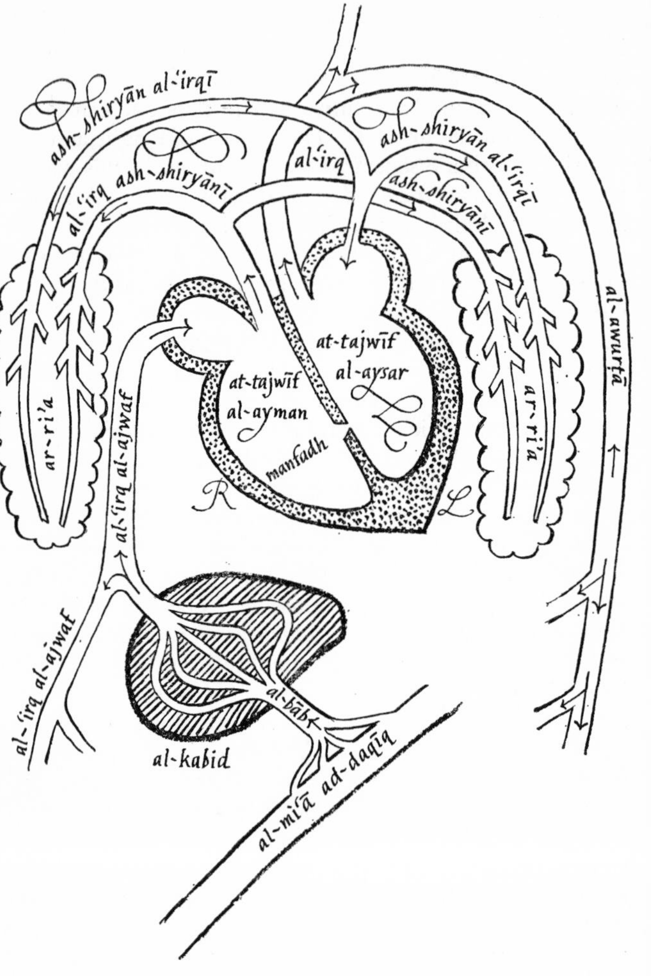

The movement of the blood
according to al-Majūsī

the anatomy and physiology of the heart and of the vessels were book-knowledge, already eight hundred years old in his time, and knowledge too which during that period had not been tested against reality because the dissection of the human body was no longer practised. Compared with Galen's account al-Majūsī's presentation again shows some simplifications and schematizations, but these cannot be gone into here.[18]

The heart is a container for the central element of life, the 'innate heat', but it was not realized that it was a mechanical pump. Arteries and veins are correctly described anatomically, but their function is conceived quite differently. The veins carry blood and also, as was seen above, the three other humours, partly as a mixture, but in addition they carry along the 'natural faculties' and the 'natural pneuma'. The arteries also contain blood, but this is finer than the venous blood. Its pure fine vapours mix with the air in the left ventricle which reaches the heart from the lungs by way of the 'venous artery'. Thus arises the 'animal pneuma' which along with the fine blood is transported through the arteries to the periphery of the body. The movement of the blood and the pneumata in the two vessel systems always goes in one direction; it is centrifugal. The blood goes from the liver by way of the vena cava and the branching veins to the periphery, and is there used in the nourishment of the organs; the fine blood and the animal pneuma reach the periphery by way of the aorta, and are there likewise used. Thus the blood in the liver and the pneuma in the heart must be constantly renewed.

A certain rather special role is played by the lungs and the vessels leading to them. Naturally the lung artery was also classified as a vein, because it comes from the right ventricle; but because its anatomical structure shows it to be an artery, it was given the compromise name of *al-ʿirq ash-shiryānī*, 'the arterial vein'. It nourishes the lungs with blood. With the vein of the lungs it is the same; it is called *ash-shiryān al-ʿirqī*, 'the venous artery', because it comes from the left ventricle but has the structure of a vein. This 'venous artery' has a double function. It transports blood and animal spirit into the lungs in order to nourish these and sustain their vital function. But it also takes air from the lungs and then passes this on to the left ventricle where it is needed to form the animal pneuma. Thus in the 'venous artery' a coming and going of different materials takes place. Such a backwards and forwards movement is not unusual. In the other arteries too a sort of 'exchange of gas' occurs, for we have seen that the arteries, when they are enlarged (namely, in the diastole), absorb the air from the heart, while in the systole they drive out the smokelike waste matter. This, be it noted, has nothing to do with the circulation of the blood as now understood, because sometimes only one vessel or one vein is in action.

The decisive thing in all this is the question of how the blood gets to the left ventricle and into the arterial system. As no communication exists between the 'arterial vein' and the 'venous artery', one must assume a passage in the septum, which guarantees the blood's flow. Galen talks of several invisible pores in the septum; al-Majūsī speaks only of one foramen, a simplification which is presumably to be blamed on the Alexandrian teaching manuals.

In the thirteenth century, the Damascus doctor 'Alā'-ad-Dīn 'Alī ibn-Abī-l-Ḥazm al-Qurashī, called Ibn-an-Nafīs,[19] takes up afresh the question of the blood's movement. Ibn-an-Nafīs, who taught medicine in Damascus and Cairo and died in 1288, wrote several commentaries on Hippocrates in which it appears he explained the material in a dry and scholarly manner. He is chiefly known for an epitome of the *Qānūn* of Ibn-Sīnā, the *Kitāb al-Mūjiz*, which was widely known as a practical handbook and was commented on by Sadīd ad-Dīn al-Kāzarūnī (d. 1357) and Nafīs ibn-'Iwaḍ al-Kirmānī (d. 1449), and in the last century was frequently lithographed and printed in India.

Ibn-an-Nafīs not only summarized the *Qānūn*, but also commented on it in a large work. Here he mentions how the blood in the right ventricle is refined so that it is prepared and ready to be mixed with the air:

> When the blood has been refined in this ventricle, it must reach the left ventricle where the pneuma (*ar-rūḥ*) is formed. But between these two ventricles there is no passage because the substance of the heart is here compact (*muṣmat*). In it there is neither a visible passage, as some suppose, nor an invisible passage which would serve to carry the blood through, as Galen thought, be-

> cause the pores (*masāmm*) of the heart are closely placed here and its substance is firm. Thus this blood, when it has been refined, must certainly reach the lungs by the arterial vein, so that it can spread out in their substance and mix with the air, so that its finest constituents can be clarified, and so that it can then reach the venous artery, and from there the left ventricle.[20]

With these words Ibn-an-Nafīs described for the first time the circulation of the lungs. But he gained his knowledge not on the basis of systematic physiological research but by plain logical deduction derived from the knowledge about the impenetrability of the septum. This must be kept in mind if the significance of his teaching is to be rightly judged. In the Islamic world this teaching has had practically no influence. Only Zayn-al-ʿArab al-Miṣrī and Sadīd-ad-Dīn al-Kāzarūnī mention it briefly.[21] On the other hand, the Spaniard Michael Servetus (Miguel Servede, 1509 – 53, in his book *Christianismi restitutio* which appeared in 1553 and which in the same year brought him to the stake in Geneva, gives a presentation of the lung circulation which resembles Ibn-an-Nafīs so strongly that one can hardly reject a direct influence. Servetus writes: 'Fit autem communicatio haec non per parietem cordis medium, ut vulgo creditur; sed magno artificio a dextro cordis ventriculo, longo per pulmones ductu, agitatur sanguis subtilis: a pulmonibus praeparatur, flavus efficitur at a vena arteriosa in arteriam venosam transfunditur'.[22] Following on Servetus, Giovanni de Valverde and Realdo Colombo, both in the middle of the sixteenth century, described the lung circulation similarly, and after another eighty years the Englishman William Harvey succeeded in 1628 in proving that the blood flows in a complete circle. But in his account too, one problem remained unexplained, namely, the transfer of the blood from the arteries into the veins. It was the microscope that first allowed Marcello Malpighi in 1661 to see the capillaries in the lungs and in the bladder of the frog. Only in this way was the last gap closed, so that the circulation of the blood was proved to be uninterrupted.

Anatomy

The anatomy of the Arabs reproduces in essentials the Galenic works *De anatomicis administrationibus* and *De anatomia ad tirones*. However, they also brought in other teachings to clear up or explain certain doubtful cases. Typical of this is the description of the human liver. Galen himself did not define exactly the number of the lobes of the liver. However, at one place in the work *De usu partium* (IV, 8) he says that the lobes of the liver encircle the stomach as with fingers. Realistically understood one could easily see the relation to the Hippocratic work *De natura ossium*,[23] where it is stated that the liver has five lobes. But as is well-known the human liver only has two lobes. Now al-Majūsī writes in his chapter on the anatomy of the stomach[24] that the liver is situated to the right of the stomach and embraces this with its five extensions (*bi-ẓawā-'idihāl-khams*). But he is more ambiguous in the chapter on the anatomy of the liver. He says that it is crescent-shaped and that its 'extensions' (*ẓawā'id*) can also be called 'extremities' (*aṭrāf*). Literally it reads: 'The liver is not uniform in all human beings but shows differences as regards its size and the number of its extremities.... The number of extremities varies; in some people there are two, others three, but in most cases there are four or five.'[25] Thus the problem here appears to have been solved by a very simple compromise, but al-Majūsī was unaware of this and instead creates a new and greater problem. He now had to explain how it is possible, in one and the same species of animal, for enormous anatomical differences to occur, and this be it noted in normal, not pathological, anatomy.

In another case, an Arab doctor succeeded in refuting an anatomical mistake of Galen's. Galen had written that the lower jaw of a human being consists of two parts, joined at the chin by a joint. The true position, however, is thus: the lower jaw in mammals is made up of two halves which in different classes of mammals fuse sooner or later and more or less firmly into a stiff symphysis in the median plane at the chin. In the higher mammals and in human beings soon after birth, the union of bones in the two halves of the chin is completed so firmly that here the lower jaw forms a single bone.

ʿAbd-al-Laṭīf al-Baghdādī had, as mentioned, made several journeys. To his stay in Egypt we are indebted for an extremely valuable book, a geographical work, in which is described the flora and fauna, the Pharaonic monuments and the typical food-stuffs, and in which he describes and discusses the problem of the Nile flood, finally giving a description of the terrible famine which befell the country in 1200–1. ʿAbd-al-Laṭīf had the opportunity in those days to see the numerous skeletons of people who had died from starvation or had been eaten by their fellows. He observes that Galen and the other doctors could scarcely have had so good an opportunity to study anatomy. At one place near Cairo a large heap of human bones lay piled. ʿAbd-al-Laṭīf counted more than two thousand skulls. When he looked at the form of the bones and joints and the way they were joined, he established that the lower jaw consists of one piece, not two, as Galen had taught. The passage that ʿAbd-al-Laṭīf refers to, occurs in chapter 6 of the book *De ossibus ad tirones*. That the lower jaw consists of two parts, says Galen, can be proved by the fact that it disintegrates at the front in the middle when 'cooked'. ʿAbd-al-Laṭīf did not think it necessary to refute this dubious proof. He opposed to it another criterion; if the lower jaw consisted of two parts connected by a joint, this joint would be visible at least in old and brittle bones, because the disintegration of the bones sets in first at the joints. With subtle irony he characterizes the great Muslim doctors as being uncritical disciples of Galen. He says: 'All are agreed that the lower jaw consists of two bones firmly joined at the chin. When I say "all", I mean by that Galen only for it is he personally who has developed the study of anatomy.'

At a time when the task of science was seen as the explanation and interpretation of tradition, not in the elaboration of something new, ʿAbd-al-Laṭīf's discovery remained without repercussions. Even if this new knowledge had not been published in such a recondite passage in a book about the geography of Egypt, it would probably have remained unnoticed. It is not mentioned in any medical work written after ʿAbd-al-Laṭīf's time. In the years that followed, the Arab doctors adhered to Galen's anatomy.[26]

FIVE

PATHOLOGY

The Aghlabid Abū-Muḍar Ziyādat-Allāh III ibn-ʿAbd-Allāh (*regnabat* 903–9) had enticed Is'ḥāq ibn-ʿImrān, who was a Muslim doctor from Baghdad despite his Jewish name, to go to Cairouan to his court by making him promises which he did not keep. Relations were strained between the doctor, who must already have been quite advanced in years, and the characterless, not very adroit ruler. Ziyādat-Allāh had Is'ḥāq's salary stopped and put him in prison. A final conversation between the two ended in a quarrel. Is'ḥāq paid for his frankness with his life. Ziyādat-Allāh had his arteries opened and bled him to death. He had the corpse crucified. It must have given satisfaction to Is'ḥāq's son ʿAlī to witness Ziyādat-Allāh's flight before the Ketama Berbers who, stirred up by Ismāʿīlī propaganda, brought about the fall of the Aghlabid dynasty in 909.

Is'ḥāq wrote a number of medical books, one of which, the treatise on melancholy, will be more fully discussed here.[1] It is of interest quite apart from the actual subject because it gives a general picture of how a certain syndrome of illness was understood, classified and explained by an Arab doctor.

The expression 'melancholy', Is'ḥāq remarks by way of introduction, denotes in fact not the illness itself but the immediate cause of the illness (*as-sabab al-adnā*), that is, black bile (*al-mirra as-sawdā'*). It is therefore a somatic illness; but it has an injurious effect upon the soul. It can be defined as 'a certain feeling of dejection and isolation which forms in the soul because of something which the patients think is real but which is in fact unreal'. The cause of the illness lies in the fact that a vapour rises from the black bile, and this presses forward to the seat of reason, dimming its light and confusing it, thus destroying the power of apprehension.

Melancholy can be innate or acquired. A person is predisposed to melancholy if his temperament (*mizāj aṣlī*) has already been injured prenatally as the result of the father's sperm having been damaged or if the mother's uterus was in a bad condition. Melancholy acquired post-natally can have the following causes: a) immoderate eating and drinking; b) neglect of the internal cleanliness of the body; c) disruption of the correct rhythms or measures of the six necessary basic presuppositions of living (*al-asbāb as-sitta al-iḍṭirāriyya*), namely, movement and rest, sleeping and waking, bowel evacuation and retention, eating and drinking, inhalation and exhalation and the soul's moods. Thus, to quote one example, too much rest and sleep lead to an accumulation of waste matter in the body, which rots and turns into black bile. But too much movement is damaging too; because of the increased heat bound up with it, the moisture in the body is used up, producing vapours which become black bile.

In addition, the following things can also produce melancholy: d) love of heavy foods which engender blood that is too hot or too dry and which quickly turns into black bile; e) living in places that are very hot and dry or cold and dry; and a stay in marshy country and sultry regions can also lead to melancholy; f) interruption of a habit, for example, of physical exercise or of regular cupping; g) drunkenness; h) asceticism, as, for example, that practised by philosophers who fast and remain awake all night. For in these cases the blood is reduced; it becomes thick and turns into black bile.

By itself, however, the excess of black bile produced by such errors does not produce melancholy. It only becomes an illness when the brain is weakened. But the weakness of the organ can come about as the result of too much heat or hypersensitivity. If both occur together, the organ attracts illness as the cupping-glass the blood.

Is'ḥāq also says that melancholy may have purely psychical causes. Fear, annoyance or anger, which appear in the 'animal soul' (*an-nafs al-ḥayawāniyya, to epithymētikon*), can encourage melancholy. So the loss of a beloved child or of an irreplaceable library can release such sadness and dejection that melancholy is the result. In the 'rational soul' (*an-nafs an-nāṭiqa, to logis-*

tikon) too, a similar process can occur: if doctors, mathematicians, or astronomers meditate, brood, memorize and investigate too much, they can fall prey to melancholy.

Is'ḥāq determines the kinds and types of melancholy in real scholarly fashion according to the categories of existence (*anniyya*), of quiddity (*māhiyya*), of quality (*kayfiyya*), and quantity (*kammiyya*). In so doing, he distinguishes three main types:

1. The first type originates in the brain itself; this melancholy is 'idiopathic'. Two subspecies must be distinguished: i) the one is accompanied by high fever; it originates in yellow bile which has only just begun to 'burn'; its symptoms are sudden movements (*tawaththub*), stupid actions (*safāha*), seeing black people. ii) the second subspecies is further divided into two: a) in the first, natural black bile is dominant in the temperament of the brain. It is called *al-waswās as-sabuʿī*, 'predator-like suggestion' because the sufferers behave like beasts of prey; b) the second subspecies originates in rotting black bile.

2. The second type comes from black bile which is released in the whole body, and which then, spreading outwards from the legs, rises to the brain. The brain is therefore 'sympathetically' affected.

3. In the third type too, the brain is 'sympathetically' affected. In this case melancholy arises because black bile takes over in the whole body and discharges itself into the upper orifice (*epigastrium*) of the stomach. The complaint is therefore localized in the hypochondria; thus it is called in Arabic *al-ʿilla ash-sharāsīfiyya*. This condition has bad effects a) on the soul and b) on the body. a) The orifice of the stomach stands, as is known, in a reciprocal relationship (*muqābala*) to the brain. The brain is therefore especially strongly exposed to the rising vapours. To this must be added the fact that the heart lies in the neighbourhood of the orifice of the stomach. But the heart provides the brain with the 'animal pneuma' which nourishes the three psychical faculties, thinking, conception and memory. But if there is an exceptional concentration of black bile near the heart, this cannot fail to influence the animal pneuma. b) The hypochondriac type of melancholy affects the body in such a way that the black bile hinders the 'digestive faculty' (*al-quwwa al-hāḍima*) in its activity. If food is not

properly digested, the illness worsens and there is a vicious circle. It is for this reason that the hypochondriac type of melancholy is so difficult to cure.

Regarding the symptoms of melancholy, the following a) psychical and b) somatic phenomena are characteristic of all three types: a) The patients are sunk in an irrational, constant sadness and dejection, in anxiety or brooding. For many, horrible pictures and forms pass before their eyes. For example, Diocles, when he was ill, saw negroes who wanted to kill him, as well as trumpeters and cymbal players who played in the corners of his room. One patient imagined that he had no head. Another's ears were ringing but this was his senses deceiving him (*ḥiss kādhib*). Yet another believed he was made of clay. A fourth disliked walking under the open sky because he thought that God, who holds the heavens, might get tired and let it fall to the ground (see p. 31 above). A characteristic symptom is for patients to demand to see a doctor urgently and to offer him all their money, and then when he comes, not to follow his advice. b) The somatic concomitants of melancholy are loss of weight and sleeplessness. Skin eruptions (*bahaq aswad* and *qawābī ṣighār*) can also appear.

The special symptoms of Type I, the sort that only occurs in the brain, are sleeplessness, headache, flickering eyes, burning hunger or, on the other hand, loss of appetite. Type II, in which the black bile rises from the legs to the brain, has the same symptoms as the first, but in addition there may also be depressions, anxiety-feelings and terror. In Type III, the hypochondriac type, there appears in particular a distended body and flatulence or a feeling of heaviness in the head. Many vomit an acid, black-bilious juice, others love solitude. Some have to weep a lot, because vapour pierces the brain. But sometimes it happens that the patients laugh a lot; in their case, the black bile is not so bad, rather their bodies possess plenty of good blood.

Finally, Is'ḥāq discusses the possibility that the melancholic may become an epileptic, an idea which appears in the *Epidemics* of Hippocrates (VI, 8, 31) and which was accepted by all ancient doctors.[2] This compelled him to produce an excursus on epilepsy. From this there follows on the second part of the book, which discusses therapy, but which we will not go into further here.

If one looks at the complete work, one is especially struck by three things. In the first place one is impressed by the clarity of presentation, by the direct and lively manner in which the individual symptoms are described. The author is trained in medicine and philosophy and has thought through his subject well. He considers the concept of melancholy in a much broader sense than does modern psychiatry. But this compels him to differentiate, and, as a result, he arrives at a subtle classification of the different types of illness. His systematic is formal and schematic but has developed logically from humoral pathology.

However, the psychogenic explanation does not fit into the system. Here, a foreign element has been introduced, which is not congruent with the theory of the humours. One must suppose that Is'ḥāq adopted this explanation because everyday experience shows that emotional shocks sometimes produce moods of depression. But perhaps in this too, Is'ḥāq is indebted to an ancient model; Aretaeus of Cappadocia[3] had already produced the psychogenic explanation.

This brings out very clearly the complete dependence of the Arab doctor on ancient authors. Is'ḥāq had an exact knowledge of Greek literature. He can even quote an obscure source like the commentary of Palladius on the *Aphorisms* of Hippocrates, in order to present a theory of laughter. He knows that the best treatise on melancholy comes from the pen of Rufus, and that Galen published no special work on this illness but treated melancholy only in the course of other writings. Is'ḥāq's presentation does in fact tally to a great extent with Galen's explanations in *De locis affectis*.[4] Galen had enumerated three types and mentions the same symptoms. It is not possible, however, to decide whether Is'ḥāq took more from Galen than from Rufus, because we cannot form an exact picture of Rufus's work since it is only preserved in fragments. Galen certainly borrowed much from Rufus, but on the other hand Rufus appears only to have known the hypochondriac type of melancholy. However that may be, the almost complete dependence of Is'ḥāq on the ancient authors is the second characteristic of this work.

The third thing that strikes one is the remoteness from reality. The delimiting of the different types of melancholy and the assigning of the different symptoms to the individual types is done purely on the basis of theoretical conjectures. The actual syndromes of illness are difficult to reconcile with the types here elaborated. The system certainly does not originate with Is'ḥāq. But one always praises the Arab doctors for the fact that they were sharp observers and acquired their own experience at the sick bed. Is'ḥāq, too, must have been able to draw on a rich source of experience. But, of this, nothing has been included in his treatise on melancholy although it was the work of his old age What Is'ḥāq gives us is learning entirely gleaned from books.

That this position is not an isolated one but typical and highly characteristic of Arab doctors is clear when one compares how, two generations later, ʿAlī ibn-al-ʿAbbās al-Majūsī understands melancholy.[5] For Majūsī too, melancholy is a sickness of the brain, for the most part somatically conditioned (that it can have psychical causes, that is, that it can arise from fright or sadness, is only mentioned casually). He, too, distinguishes between the idiopathic and the sympathetic course of the illness. In the first, the brain itself is sick, in the second, it is either the black bile vapours which rise from the stomach to the brain, or it is the burnt-up humours of the whole body that affect the brain (he calls this kind *al-ʿilla al-marāqqiyya wa-n-nāfikha, to nosēma hypokhondriakon kai physōdes*, cf. Galen, VIII, 185).

This last type is subdivided by al-Majūsī into three parts and here he differs basically from Is'ḥāq ibn-ʿImrān: a) the first type arises from the blood; the confusion of the reason expresses itself in euphoria, in laughing and jollity; this form is tied up with a certain type of constitution: the patients are thinner, have very hairy chests, their skin colouring is brown to red, their veins are large, the pulse beats strongly but slowly. b) The second type arises because yellow bile is 'burnt' in the body; the patients have a wavering gaze, they make mischief, they scream, are prone to angry outbursts and are troubled with restlessness and sleeplessness. c) The third type is the result of black bile; the patients are given over to cares, broodings, anxieties and evil imaginings. Many love solitude. Thus al-Majūsī reduces the different types of melancholy to the humours, but does not consider the phlegm as a possible cause of illness. Yet, even in so doing, he introduces nothing new. The distinction of types according to the humours, with the characteristic exception of the phlegm, comes from Alexander of Tralles.[6]

In a second point, too, al-Majūsī differs from Is'ḥāq's conception: he reckons lycanthropy likewise to be a form of melancholy, without however assigning a place to it in the system already developed. He cannot do this because he has nothing to say about its aetiology. The sick man imitates hens or dogs; at night he wanders about the cemeteries. His skin is yellow, his eyes appear dark and sunken, his mouth is dry and lacking in saliva, he has scratch marks and bite marks on his legs as well as ulcers. Lycanthropy is as good as incurable. The basis of this syndrome is the old belief in the werwolf; Marcellus of Side gave this popular belief a medical interpretation, and for obvious reasons reckoned it to be a form of melancholy. Galen knew nothing of it but Oribasius (*Synopsis*, VIII, 9), Aetius of Amida (VI, 11) and Paul of Aegina (III, 16) took over Marcellus's interpretation and in this way the Arabs learnt about lycanthropy. Thus it happens that al-Majūsī's syndrome agrees with that of the Byzantine compilers in every detail; indeed, even the Arabic name for the illness, *al-quṭrub*, is only a clumsy reproduction of the Greek word *lykanthropia*.

In this way, nearly all the ideas produced by the Arab authors about melancholy go back to ancient sources. Ibn-Sīnā represents essentially the same concept as al-Majūsī, but in other presentations, for example, in the *Kitāb adh-Dhakhīra* ascribed to Thābit ibn-Qurra, theory retreats completely behind practical therapeutic advice. The most famous ancient theory, however, that of Theophrastus, was, as far as I can see, not seized upon by the Arab doctors. Theophrastus's work on melancholy is preserved as an excerpt in the pseudo-Aristotelian *Problemata physica*, and the *Problemata* have also been translated into Arabic under the title *Kitāb Mā bāl*. The Arabs were thus fully aware of Theophrastus's thesis that genial people are melancholic, that thesis which leads on to the general problem of 'genius and madness'. But the question was medically irrelevant. Certainly the Arab authors who wrote about melancholy fulfilled to the utmost Galen's demand that every doctor must be a philosopher. But the contents of their medical and their philosophical thinking continued to follow each its own course. Here, there were scarcely any cross-relationships; rather the authors remained caught in preconceived models of thinking.

The adherence to tradition in pathological teaching can once again be well demonstrated in the case of diabetes. According to al-Majūsī,[7] diabetes occurs because of the too great strength of the 'attractive faculty', by which the kidneys attract the watery constituents of the blood, in other words, the urine. Thus the cause lies in a hot dyscrasy of the kidneys which consequently need the water to extinguish and cool the flaming heat (*lahīb*) present in them. Thus they attract away the moisture from the liver and the other organs, so that the person experiences a burning thirst. A second possibility for the occurrence of diabetes lies in the weakness of the 'retentive faculty' of the kidneys which cannot retain in themselves the watery constituents reaching them from the liver. One can diagnose diabetes by the following signs: the patient feels a burning thirst though there is no fever, nor is the body dried out; he produces urine constantly without this burning; the urine is thin, pale, and resembles water because the water that the patient drinks immediately passes out as urine without it being able to undergo change in the liver.

Al-Majūsī's presentation, which coincides with Galen's explanations,[8] is extremely brief and scanty, but fortunately we have a monograph on diabetes, a *Consilium* by ʿAbd-al-Laṭīf al-Baghdādī.[9] Right at the beginning, ʿAbd-al-Laṭīf speaks of the 'aforesaid patient' and later he again mentions 'this patient', but not by name. It is therefore a confidential opinion written only for colleagues who were personally concerned with the case. A patient who could collect several doctors around him must have been a high-placed personage. An allusion at a later point helps us further. ʿAbd-al-Laṭīf there defines his attitude vis-à-vis a doctor, 'a man from the Maghrib, an old man in years but a child in knowledge and insight', and refutes the latter's views. By this colleague he meant the same Maghribi sheikh against whom he polemicized in his *Kitāb an-Naṣīḥatayn*,[10] namely, Abū-l-Ḥajjāj Yūsuf ibn-Yaḥyā ibn-Shamʿūn, the favourite pupil of Maimonides. Abū-l-Ḥajjāj had to flee from Fez because of persecution by the Almohads; he settled in Aleppo and was one of the doctors present at the death in 1216 of al-Malik aẓ-Ẓāhir Ghāzī ibn-Yūsuf, a son of Saladin. Since in this expert opinion on diabetes it is particularly mentioned that the question at issue was discussed 'at the court of the sultan' and since ʿAbd-al-Laṭīf lived in Aleppo from 1216 to 1220, the same historical framework can be presumed. The expert opinion was therefore written in 1216 and the patient was none other than Ghāzī ibn-Yūsuf.

According to ʿAbd-al-Laṭīf's view, diabetes consists in 'polyuria' for which there are four causes: 1) a weakness or paralysis of the sphincter of the bladder; 2) a piercing pain in the urinary passages; 3) a weakness in the 'retentive faculty' of the kidneys; 4) a hot dyscrasy of the kidneys. The third and fourth points are already known to us from al-Majūsī's book; the first and second rather dispense with logic because these complaints may result in urinary discharge but not necessarily in polyuria. Nevertheless, it must be recognized that ʿAbd-al-Laṭīf wanted to present diabetes as comprehensively as possible. What he gives us are quite heterogeneous syndromes, but the most important symptoms of diabetes, namely, the raised sugar content and the sweet taste of the urine, were known neither to him, nor to al-Majūsī, nor to Ibn-Sīnā.

This is a little surprising for, in support of his view, ʿAbd-al-Laṭīf quotes, inter alia, longer passages from the *Kitāb al-Ḥāwī* of ar-Rāzī, and precisely in this work there are two passages where the examination of urine in respect of taste is discussed. One of the passages comes from a writing by Rufus and reads: 'When examining urine, one must be careful to note the amount, whether little or great, its colour, its taste, its smell, its consistency, that is, whether thick or thin.'[11] The other passage comes from the anonymous book, *Kitāb ad-Dalāʾil*, an ancient work on diagnosis: 'In the case of urine, three things must be examined, its colour, its consistency, and its sediment. In addition, its smell, its temperature when a finger is placed in it, and its pungency of taste should be tested.'[12] That the testing of urine by the tongue was not unknown to the Arabs is also seen from a poem in which Ibn-al-Munajjim mocks the Jewish doctor Hibat-Allāh ibn-Jumayʿ: 'He cannot determine the urine of a sick man in the glass, not even when he rolls it on the tongue.' One may well ask whether this method, which is not pleasant for the doctor, was in fact practised. But the truth is that no Arab mentions the sweet taste of a diabetic's urine. In their knowledge of this illness, the Arabs have not left the Greeks behind.

The adoption of Greek medicine by the Arabs meant the introduction of a certain canon of clinical syndromes in countries in which, on account of their geographical position, other illnesses are also endemic. At first there appears to be no very great difference, for the medicine of the Hellenistic and imperial periods and of later antiquity was, above all, carried on by doctors who practised in Asia Minor, Syria and Egypt – in fact, in those very countries which were later to belong to the heartlands of Islam. But Greek medicine was also current in the Arabian peninsula, in Iraq, Persia, Transoxania, Afghanistan, and in large parts of North Africa and Spain, in regions therefore in which illnesses prevailed which the Greeks had described either not at all or not satisfactorily. It must therefore be asked whether the Arab doctors were in a position, given the theoretical equipment and the concepts of diagnosis and nosology left them by the Greeks, to describe new illnesses or only to comprehend more precisely illnesses only incompletely known. Were they indeed conscious of the fact that it was possible and necessary to add something to the 'perfect' Greek system?

Enlightening is the case of the guinea-worm, also called the Medina-worm (*Dracunculus medinensis*), a parasite which attacks human beings. The female worm is generally a metre long and lives subcutaneously in the tissue. On maturity, the head of the worm breaks through the skin (preferably of the lower extremities) and discharges large numbers of larvae (*microfilaria*) into stagnant water. There the larvae are eaten by Cyclops-crabs, and by way of drinking water contaminated by these crabs reach the human stomach where they lodge themselves. The worm needs about a year to reach full maturity. It can be extracted at the point of breakthrough.[13]

In ancient times, this cycle was naturally not yet known. Galen had only heard from many people that in a place in Arabia there were 'little snakes' (*drakontia*) that had a 'nerve-like' nature similar to intestinal worms in colour and thickness. He says that he himself has never seen them and can therefore say nothing exactly either about their origin or their nature.[14] But before Galen, Leonidas and Soranus had written about the *drakontia* as Paul of Aegina reports.[15] Soranus had disputed the animal nature of this illness, rather he took it to be a nerve. We read similarly in the post-classical anonymous *Book of Signs* (*Kitāb al-ʿĀlāmāt*) which we only know from one Arabic source: 'The illness arises because a nerve (*ʿaṣab*) disintegrates; thus one gets the impression that the thing is moving'.[16] And also in the pseudo-Galenic *Definitiones medicae* (no. 437)[17] the *drakontion* is designated a 'nerve'. Paulus himself gives no clear explanation. So when in the Arab authors the illness constantly bears the name *al-ʿirq al-madanī*, 'the Medinan vein', it may be due to the influence of the pseudo-Galenic work *Introductio seu medicus* in which in chapter XIX[18] we read that the so-called *drakontia* resemble 'varicose veins' (*kirsoi*). At any rate, the knowledge that this had to do with a parasitosis, an infestation, was thus terminologically barred for the Arabs. Their awareness that the illness is endemic in the Hejaz caused them to call this 'vein' 'Medinan'.

The great encyclopaedias, of al-Majūsī[19] and az-Zahrāwī,[20] only reproduced what Paul of Aegina had already said. However, ʿAbd-Allāh ibn-Yaḥyā, a doctor of the ninth century, goes beyond the ancient author when in his *Kitāb al-Ikhtiṣārāt*[21] he writes that the Medinan vein occurs in hot countries and is the result of drinking bad water. It develops as the result of hot phlegm that has become sharp.[22] The theory that it arises from phlegm was clearly held by Qusṭā ibn-Lūqā, for he writes in his *Book on Phlegm*: 'In Samarra I once saw a man in whose body forty veins had formed but he got rid of all of them.'[23]

If the Arabs could bring nothing new in the way of theory, they did, however, present some interesting clinical reports. In this connection, ar-Rāzī in particular communicates his discoveries: 'In the hospital, I saw a thing that was torn off. Then we opened the place up, though without even troubling to look for the "vein", but opened up the wound correctly with the finger. Then we treated it and it healed completely.'[24] Ar-Rāzī goes on: 'The nephew of al-Huṣayn ibn-ʿAdawayh has told me that he suffered with the Medinan vein and it was cut up more than once. Then a man from the Hejaz instructed him that he ought to take a half drachm of aloes for three days. This

مشبه المنفصل له اسنان في الطرف كاترى وقد يصنع مستطيلة

كالكلاليب عليه هذه الصور كاترى لها اسنان كاسنان المنشار يقطع

بها وينفصل ن شاء الله تعالى

صورة مدفع ايضًا

صورة صنان

هذه الصنان فيها غلظ قليلا ليلا يسكر عند جذب الجنين بها

صورة صنان ذات الشوكتين

صورة مبضعين عريضين لقطع الجنين

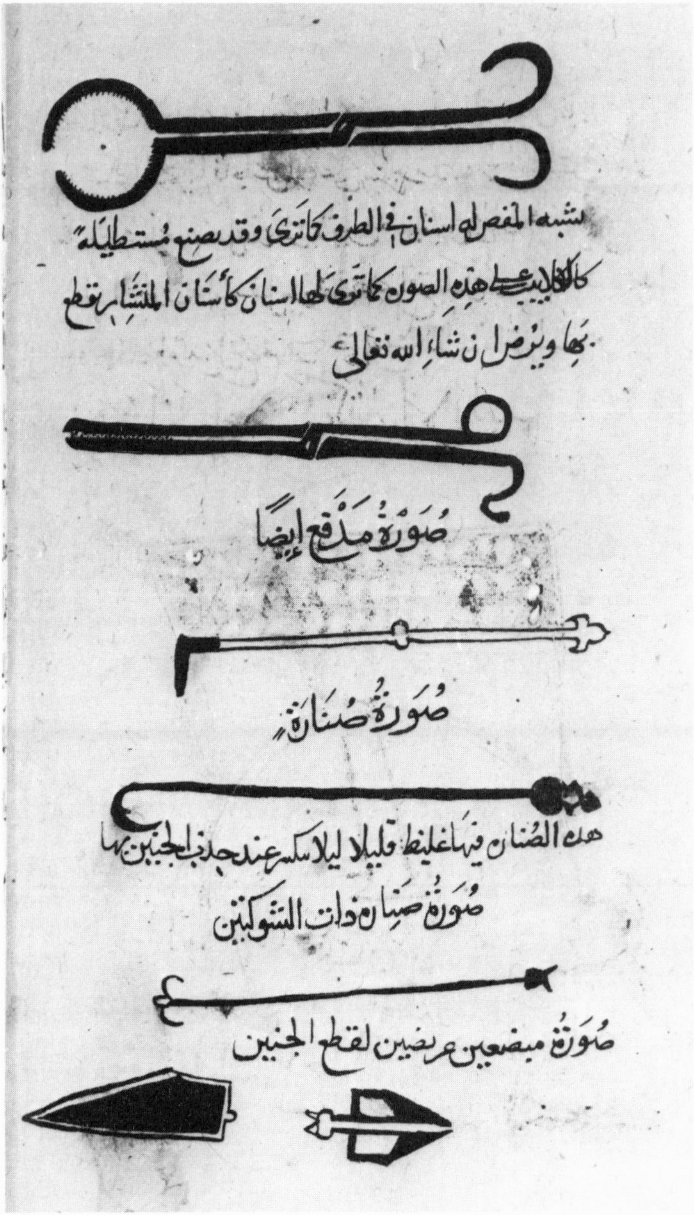

PLATE 5. Some chirurgical instruments, according to
Abū-l-Qāsim az-Zahrāwī

PLATE. 6 An Arab pharmacy, from a Dioscurides MS

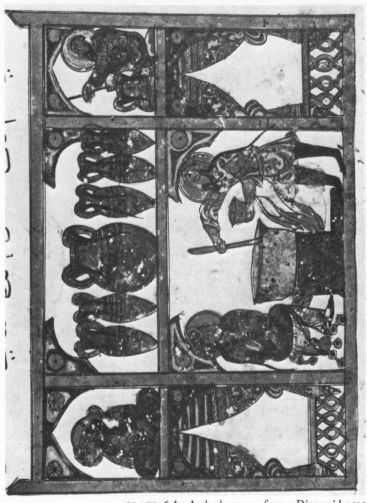

he did, and immediately the pain stopped. Neither then nor at a later date up to the present time has anything emerged.' Ar-Rāzī adds by way of explanation: 'This man had a warm temperament, large veins, was very hirsute and muscular.'[25] That ar-Rāzī thought the patient's constitution worthy of note is shown in a further opinion: 'I have noticed that the Medinan vein practically never comes out if bodies have wet flesh; but in muscular or lean physiques it comes out. Nor does it come out in those who visit the bath regularly, go into the water, drink wine and eat well.'[26]

These reports and observations are without doubt good. But this does not mean that the Arabs, because of their more exact knowledge of local conditions and the frequency of the appearance of the illness in their countries, could have described the illness itself more exactly or could have revised the account given by Paul. They were not even aware of the animal nature of the illness. Ibn-Sīnā[27] states expressly: 'Sometimes it makes a worm-like movement under the skin, as if it were the movement of an animal and as if the illness was in truth a worm. Yes, there are people who imagine it is an animal that has grown [in the body].' It was only the German doctor and orientalist, Engelbert Kaempfer (1651–1716) who in 1683 made long journeys in the East and who gave a very exact description of the worm, the way to draw it out and its beginnings as the result of drinking foul rain-water (naturally he did not know the intermediate host, *Cyclops*). But he does not forget to polemicize against Rhazes and Avicenna who mistook the type of parasite and designated the worm a 'vein' or a 'nerve'.[28]

There is proof, too, of ar-Rāzī's clinical acuteness in the case of smallpox. Smallpox was not described, or was not sufficiently described, by the ancient doctors. Apart from brief mentions of the illness in the 'Presbyter Ahrun' and in ʿAlī ibn-Sahl aṭ-Ṭabarī, the *Kitāb al-Judarī wa-l-ḥaṣba* (*De variolis et morbillis*) of ar-Rāzī is the first work in which the illness is fully treated and in which its symptoms are described. The illness is ultimately produced from the impurity of the blood of the child arising from bad menstrual blood which was not got rid of during the pregnancy. At puberty, these materials begin to boil up in the same way as wine ferments, and pockmarks form as a result. Ar-Rāzī writes:

> The outbreak of smallpox is preceded by constant fever, back pains, itchy nose and uneasiness in sleep. These are the specific symptoms of its onset: in particular, back pains accompanied by fever; then a stinging feeling through the patient's whole body; a swelling of the face, sometimes a wasting-away of the same; flushing of the skin; violent crimson of the cheeks; redness of the eyes; heaviness in the whole body; pain in the throat and chest combined with a certain difficulty in breathing; dryness of the mouth and thick saliva; roughness of the voice; headaches; heaviness in the head; restlessness, bad temper, nausea, dejection; (but restlessness, nausea and dejection are more commonly met with in measles than in smallpox, while back pains are especially typical of smallpox, not of measles); heat in the whole body; flushing and redness of the skin; and, in particular, the gums are inflamed.

Al-Majūsī,[29] like ar-Rāzī, sees the ultimate cause of smallpox in the menstrual blood which has nourished the foetus. If the foul remainder of this blood remains in its organs and veins, it breaks out later in the form of pockmarks. The description of the different forms of smallpox is, however, so imprecise that modern research has identified it with erysipelas, chickenpox (Varicellae), genuine smallpox, anthrax and measles.[30]

It appears that in one case we are indebted to ar-Rāzī, the clinician, for the description of a really 'new' syndrome: the fact that the scent of roses for certain sensitive people produces an allergic cold or catarrh was only described relatively late in medical literature. In the sixteenth and seventeenth centuries a few cases were registered in Europe and, in the nineteenth century, American and English authors like Morill Wyman (1872) and Morell Mackenzie (1884) described further cases under the designation 'rose-cold' or 'rose-fever'.[31] But ar-Rāzī had already written an expert opinion on the illness, which afflicted the founder of classical Arabic geography, Abū-Zayd Aḥmad ibn-Sahl al-Balkhī, every spring when the roses bloomed. In it he says quite plainly that it is the rose-scent that causes the cold and he recommends the patient to avoid smelling things that give off a lot of vapours, for example, roses, the small basil herb, fish, onions, leeks, garlic and wine. Apart from this, his advice follows the conventional pattern: the patient should not sleep in damp rooms and caves, he should not go bare-headed in cold weather, etc. In urgent cases, cupping of the neck cavity and bleeding of the temple arteries are advocated.[32]

Real progress was made by the Arabs in the description of the plague, and this will be more fully discussed in the following chapter. In general one can say that a man like ar-Rāzī made excellent observations, but he did not arrive at any new theoretical foundations or a more exact grasp of the essence of an illness. Spectacular illnesses endemic in the East, like bilharziasis in Egypt, did not attract the attention of the Arab doctors. The syndromes which Galen and the post-classical authors handed down remained for the Arabs, too, paradigms of their medical activity.

SIX

THE TRANSMISSIBILITY OF ILLNESSES AND THE PLAGUE

It was obviously assumed in ancient times that illnesses are transmissible but the transmissibility was not yet conceived or formulated as a general principle. In his account of the plague at Athens in 430 B.C., Thucydides speaks quite naturally of infection – through nursing, one infects the other – and he also knows about immunity when someone has survived an illness. He says: 'It does not attack the same person twice, at least not fatally.' When the plague arrived in 166, Galen fled from Rome. Galen[1] also speaks of the danger of being in contact with sufferers from plague (*tois loimōttusin*) because there exists the danger that one becomes infected as in the case of scab (*psōra*) or trachoma (*ophthalmia*) or consumption (*phthoē*), or all the illnesses that produce bad breath.

In ancient Arabia, the transmission of illnesses was similarly assumed as a matter of course. Al-Ḥārith ibn-Ḥilliza al-Yashkurī suffered from leprosy (*waḍaḥ*). When he was to recite his Muʿallaqa before ʿAmr ibn-Hind, king of al-Ḥīra, ʿAmr ordered a screen to be placed between them.[2] An-Nābigha adh-Dhubyānī (ed. Fayṣal no. LXXV, 37) complains: 'There I spent the night as though I were an outcast, a condemned person whom people have driven away, or a severely ill person, suffering from plague (*taʿīn*).' The bedouin especially made the discovery that mange in camels (*jarab*) is infectious. Al-Muzarrid (VIII, 3) says: 'I was like one who exchanged a perfectly healthy camel for a mangy camel which infects him who comes into contact with her'; and in Dhū r-Rumma (LX, 4) we read: 'Like a mangy camel smeared with tar and isolated in a desert place so that other camels do not come into contact with her.'

The early Islamic community had the same idea as is shown

by the Ḥadīth, those teachings which ostensibly go back to the prophet Muḥammad. There we read, for example, 'The owner of sick animals should not drive these to the owner of healthy animals', and in another passage is written, 'Fly from the leper (*al-majdhūm*) as you would fly from a lion.' Also the saying, 'If you hear that plague has broken out in a country, do not go there; if it breaks out in a country where you are staying, do not leave it',[3] is presumably meant to be interpreted that the inhabitants of a plague-infested place should suffer sickness and death rather than endanger the inhabitants of other healthy places by taking the plague there. In this last saying experiences from a recurrence of the Justinian plague may have left their mark. Another enigmatic and verbally obscure saying roused feelings and led to endless discussion which has lasted to the present day:[4] *lā ʿadwā wa-lā ṭiyarata wa-lā hāmata wa-lā ṣafara.*[5] A possible translation would be: 'There is no transmission, no augury, no bird of death (owl) and no . . .' (the meaning of the last word is unknown). It is clear that this saying was directed against heathen divination practices still in use at that time and it is very questionable whether the word *ʿadwā* here is used especially in the sense of 'transmission of illnesses'. Despite this, the theological discussion has so understood the word, has taken it out of its apparent context, and from it has deduced the dogma that according to the prophet's teaching there is no infection.[6]

In the medical works written by the Arabs since the ninth century and based on Greek sources infection is discussed. The doctors speak of *iʿdā'* and in so doing, they are naturally not making a conceptual distinction between infection (direct transmission of bacilli) and contagion (transmission of parasites and the like). The word *iʿdā'* is even used when one is talking about hereditary illness so that one is best to translate quite generally by 'transmission' or 'transmissibility'. This conceptual breadth or lack of precision clearly finds an expression in al-Majūsī when he describes elephantiasis (*judhām*).[7] It rests on a cold and dry dyscrasy and on the circumstance that the black-bilious (*al-khilṭ as-sawdāwī*) humour is dominant in the blood and breaks it up. Since the semen originates from the blood, the corruption spreads also to it so that this illness is transmitted to future generations (*ḥattā inna hādhihi l-ʿillata tuʿdī n-nasla*) and reappears in the children. Taken literally, it is as if the substance of the semen has got mixed with the bad humours which produce this illness. The humours of the child that has originated from this semen are in similar condition to those humours, and its basic organs grow out of their substance. Consequently this illness is transmitted by the parents to the children (*tataʿaddā*). It is significant that al-Majūsī continues by using the same idea: 'Sometimes this illness is transmitted (*yataʿaddā*) to one sitting near the patients and talking with them, because an evil vapour (*bukhār radī*) comes from their bodies which the one standing nearest them inhales.'

In another passage,[8] al-Majūsī gives a small catalogue of 'transmissible illnesses' (*amrāḍ muʿdiya*). He includes leprosy or elephantiasis (*judhām*), scab (*jarab*), consumption (*sill*), phrenitis (*birsām*), smallpox (*judarī*), trachoma (*ramad*), and strangely enough, also albugo (*Pterygium, sabal*). A similar catalogue occurs in the *Kitāb adh-Dhakhīra* ascribed to Thābit ibn-Qurra. According to this, leprosy or elephantiasis, scab, smallpox, measles (*ḥaṣba*), ozaena (*bakhar*), trachoma and the various forms of plague (*al-amrāḍ al-wabāʾiyya*) are infectious.

The more magically oriented authors show as little doubt about infection. They place this in the area of 'sympathetic effects' (*khawāṣṣ*) and thereby avoid the need to give an explanation for the phenomenon. Al-Qazwīnī,[9] who reproduces older sources, writes:

> The 'hidden movement' (*sirāya*) of certain illnesses also belongs to the sympathetic effects. It is thus asserted that to gaze constantly at a trachomatic eye (*al-ʿayn ar-ramida*) will necessarily lead to the illness being transmitted to the one gazing. If one eats what has been left by someone with scab, phrenitis, elephantiasis, leprosy or diphtheria (*khunāq*), this will lead to the transmission of the illness. If a leper walks barefoot over the soil, plants will no longer grow in those places where his feet trod.

'Transmission' (*iʿdā*) can also happen when according to our ideas, there is no infective illness present: when at ʿAskar Mukram or Gondēshāpūr a man was stung by a scorpion (*jarrāra*) and killed, it came about that his flesh fell from his bones; or it decayed and stank so badly that one only approached the corpse after covering one's nose with a mask for fear of transmission (*makhāfata iʿdāʾi-hī*).[10] Transmission therefore results from fetid air and through a miasma, and from this the concept is named which has played a decisive role in the theory of transmission of plague since Hippocrates.

However no exact nosography of the plague appears in classical Islam (ninth to twelfth century) as can be shown from the following theory reported by al-Majūsī:[11] the air loses its uniform, normal composition (*iʿtidāl*). Its substance and qualities are turned into decay and putrefaction so that many bad illnesses appear simultaneously in people, for example, confused reason, pains, sweatings, cold of the extremities, burning in the breast, dryness and bad taste in the mouth, thirst, spasms in the hypochondria, bilious vomitings and bilious diarrhoea, meteorism, bad urine etc.[12] These complaints are called 'epidemic illnesses' (*amrāḍ wāfida*) because they affect many people at the same time. Their cause is in fact the air surrounding us. Their worsening may have a local and a temporal cause.

The local cause consists of bad vapours or exhalations (*bukhārāt*) which rise up from masses of putrefying fruits and plants and mix with the air. These exhalations can come from ditches, stagnant waters and marshes, from the garbage of towns, from soldiers fallen on the battlefield, from dead bodies of animals fallen prey to pestilence. When human beings inhale this putrid air, they fall prey to corrupting illnesses (in this passage, though al-Majūsī does not say so, it is assumed that the inhaled air becomes a part of the 'animal pneuma' which passes through the arteries to all the organs). So it was with the Athenians who were visited by death when the evil vapours of the men who died in Ethiopia reached them.[13]

The temporal cause consists of the fact that certain seasons of the year are, contrary to their real nature, unnaturally hot, dry, rainy, or cold, for example, heat in winter. This results in death, plague (*wabāʾ*), pestilence (*ṭawāʿīn*), smallpox (*judarī*), high fever, etc. The baneful circumstances can even affect cattle and plants, and whoever eats such dry and dusty plants also falls ill.

In all this, however, the predisposition of men is of decisive importance. The putrid air by itself does not engender pestilential illnesses; these occur rather in those whose bodies have already assembled bad and corrupt humours. It is the convergence (*mushākala*) of both factors that leads to the growth of corrupting illnesses. Bodies which have no waste matter, that is, such as those whose health is well cared for, remain spared the above-mentioned illnesses. If it were not so, everyone would sicken at once with plague and succumb. This view of predisposition (*isti'dād*) has, according to al-Majūsī, been stressed by Galen in his book *De differentiis febrium.*[14]

In the practical section of his book,[15] al-Majūsī deals briefly with the miasmata and the predisposition so as to recommend prophylactic measures against the epidemic illnesses: one must follow a way of life which counterbalances the mixture which the air has at that time, one must empty out the bodily humour which has a similar form to the mixture of the air, whether it be by bleeding or by an emptying of the bowels which will take away the hot waste matter; one should not expose one's self to the hot sun and the hot winds but seek refreshment in cool places, inhabit dwellings facing north, scatter myrtle and roses in them, fumigate them with camphor and sandalwood, etc. As medicaments are offered 'Armenian earth' (*hē ek tēs Armenias bōlos*, *aṭ-ṭīn al-armanī*),[16] camphor pastilles, and other drugs.

Two things are particularly striking about this chapter: the blurring of ideas and the absence of precise nosography.

The chapter is headed 'prophylaxis against pestilential illnesses' (*al-amrāḍ al-wabā'iyya*) which are identical with the 'epidemic illnesses' (*al-amrāḍ al-wāfida*) of Hippocrates. These are the illnesses 'which reach the body from outside' (*al-wārida 'alā l-badan min khārij*). For example, the 'pestilential illnesses' or 'bubonic plague' (*aṭ-ṭawā'īn*), the 'evil, death-bringing fevers' (*al-ḥummayāt al-khabītha al-muhlika*) and smallpox (*judarī*) are mentioned. But smallpox, along with leprosy, scab, etc. is also listed with the 'infectious illnesses' at the end of the chapter (see above, p. 88). The concept *i'dā'* 'transmissibility' is used here unreflectively. Everything that al-Majūsī had enumerated under 'pestilential' illnesses rests largely on *i'dā'*, and in the case of pestilential illnesses it was expressly stated that 'they reach the body from outside' which cannot but mean that they were transmitted.

The second thing that strikes one about al Majūsī's presentation is the fact that the 'plague', that extremely dramatic epidemic illness of the Middle Ages, is only mentioned casually, that it is named along with 'evil fevers', smallpox, and other illnesses as an example of 'epidemic' illnesses. One would have expected that al-Majūsī would have given over a special chapter to such a spectacular and dangerous fever and would have given a full description of its symptoms. Nothing about all this. This can only be explained by the fact that the 'plague of Justinian', that pandemic which first appeared in Pelusium in 541 and flared up again several times until the middle of the eighth century, occurred during a 'dead' period in medical literature. Galen's book *De differentiis febrium* had been written before 180, and the medical literature of the Arabs had not yet begun. The Byzantine doctors were compilers who copied only the authors of the classical, Hellenistic and imperial periods, Galen above all. Only in Oribasius is there a superb description of the bubonic plague according to Rufus of Ephesus, but this passage was obviously not known to the Arab doctors.[17] So al-Majūsī could not know more about the plague in principle than what Galen had written in his book *De differentiis febrium*. He did not take any note of the theological discussion about the Ḥadīth *lā ʿadwā*. That this theological discussion remained without any practical consequences is seen in the prescription that the market overseer (*muḥtasib*) must not allow people suffering from leprosy or elephantiasis to visit the bath.[18]

Things only acquire a different aspect when the second pandemic, the Black Death of 1348, breaks out in the Mediterranean countries.[19] It is that event which Boccaccio describes so movingly in the introduction to his *Decamerone*, and which as a result found its way into world literature. The horrifying experiences of mass dying compelled people to observe the plague afresh and independently. Thus in contemporary accounts both positions, that of the theologians and that of the doctors, are defended. The struggle which took place in the nineteenth century between the 'bacteriologists' and the 'anti-contagionists' had its prelude here, and there is no reason for us to suppose that the Muslim theologians of the fourteenth century were struck with blindness after we learn that the anti-contagionists, under the leadership of Rudolf Virchow, denied the contagious character of yellow fever, plague, cholera, leprosy and influenza, and denied the idea of a *contagium vivum*, a living disease germ.[20]

Shortly before Abū-Ḥafṣ ʿUmar ibn-Muẓaffar ibn-ʿUmar al-Wardī died of plague in 1349 in his home town Aleppo, he wrote an account in which he describes how the plague arose in Central Asia, made its way over the Crimea and spread into Palestine and Syria. He knows of no cure but he finds comfort in religion. He who dies of plague will be deemed a martyr and so become worthy of Paradise. For him, there is no transmission of the illness. It is God who creates the plague ever anew (*yubdi'u wa-yuʿīdu*). With the words of the Prophet in mind, Ibn-al-Wardī refuses to fly from the plague-stricken city.[21]

The three Spanish authors who in 1348 published treatises about the plague thought rather differently. Muḥammad ibn-al-Lakhmī ash-Shaqūrī (that is, from Segura) wrote a little book of which only an abridgement by himself has been preserved.[22] He sides with the theologians but stresses the need for medical measures. The cause of the plague is the impurity of the air, because of which lung-sufferers especially must be on their guard. Therefore the air must be improved by fumigations with *sandarak*, incense, styrax, myrrh etc. The dwelling must be freshly ventilated and the sunlight must have access. The body must be kept clean by suitable nourishment and medicine. One should avoid visiting public baths. Blood-letting should only be undertaken on the specific advice of the doctor, and similarly one should only take drugs prescribed by the doctor. That magic also plays a role in medical measures is natural for that time; the carrying of a hyacinth can ward off the plague and if one hangs the piece of a tusk of the elephant round a child's neck, he is secure against the plague.[23]

We have to thank two other authors, the writer Aḥmad ibn-ʿAlī ibn-Muḥammad ibn-Khātima (d. *c.* 1369) and the statesman and historian, Lisān-ad-Dīn ibn-al-Khaṭīb,[24] for exact descriptions of the symptoms of the plague. Ibn-al-Khaṭīb also published other medical works, for example, the *Kitāb ʿAmal man ṭabba*, a general pathology,[25] and the *Kitāb al-Wuṣūl*, a book on hygiene, both extremely dry and unoriginal compilations. One is all the more surprised at the directness and freshness of the presentation which he follows in his writing on the plague, the *Kitāb Muqniʿat as-sā'il*.[26] Ibn-al-Khaṭīb teaches:

When the illness enters the body of a man through transmission and contagion (*intiqālan wa-ʿadwā*), which is generally the case, the pneuma is influenced by it, sometimes immediately, but sometimes only after the body has built up a resistance according to predisposition. Then the body gets hot, and fever ensues which circulates in the arteries. Now the juices in the veins (*ruṭūbāt*) become corrupt, the blood boils because it tries to drive out the corrupt juices. If the nature is up to this task and is supported by lunar and spherical conditions (as taught by those who busy themselves with 'crises'), it drives out the juices with the help of the 'crises' and in the well-known ways, namely, in urine, stools, sweat, nose-bleedings or other haemorrhages. In this manner, improvement sets in. If the nature does not have so much strength, it drives the juices to the places to which the morbid material of the cardinal organs has been pushed, namely, the cavities behind the ears, under the armpits, and at the appendage of the upper thigh (the lymphatic nodes). If they settle here and if there is still some resistance present, the corrupt juices are enclosed at these points. The 'innate heat' (*al-ḥārr al-gharīzī*) attacks them in order to curb the poisonous matter and to resolve it by 'cooking' (*inḍāj*). In this way, recovery sets in. But if the nature is not equal to the poisonous material, it becomes feeble and evil signs and fatal crises set in. These materials are transported to the place which offers least resistance to the evil, and that is the lung because of its loose structure, its movement, its passivity and its predisposition if it is exposed from the beginning to the inhalation of the poison. It swells, and we see symptoms of inflammation of the lungs (*dhāt ar-ri'a*); because of their nearness the organs of the thorax also break down and we get the spitting up of blood. If there is still some power of resistance in the nature, the materials are pushed back to the three places mentioned, or elsewhere, after they had nearly settled in the lungs and some symptoms had made themselves noticeable. But the lung can no longer recover. The force of the poison is renewed behind it so that it conquers and extinguishes the vital spirit (the pneuma). Sometimes visible swellings remain, sometimes the places collapse. In this way, death occurs.

Ibn-al-Khaṭīb stresses that his presentation of the course of the illness is in agreement with medical art and that examination has shown this, after taking into consideration the anatomical and other presuppositions. He now explains the idea of predisposition according to Galen, in order then to be able to speak about the transmissibility of the plague:

> If one asks, 'How can you admit the assertion, there is infection, when the revealed word (*ash-shar'*) denies this?' we answer: that infection exists, is confirmed by experience, research, insight and observation and through constantly recurring accounts. These are the elements of proof. For him who has treated or recognized this case, it cannot remain concealed that mostly the man who has had contact with a patient infected with this disease must die, and that, on the other hand, the man who has had no contact remains healthy. So it is with the appearance of the illness in a house or quarter because of a garment or a vessel; even an earring can destroy him who puts it in his ear, and all the inhabitants of the house. The illness can first appear in a town in a single house; then, from there, it can break out among individual contacts, then among their neighbours, relatives, and especially their visitors, until the breach becomes even greater. The illness can appear in coastal towns that enjoyed good health until there lands in them a man with plague, come from across the sea, from another coast where the plague already exists, as reports tell. The date of the appearance of the illness in the town tallies with the date of debarcation of this man. Many remained healthy who kept themselves strictly cut off from the outside world, like the pious Ibn-Abī-Madyan in Salé. He belonged to those who believed in contagion. He had stored up provisions for a long period and bricked up his door behind him and his large family. The town succumbed but during that period, he was not deprived of a single soul. One had repeatedly heard that places which lie remote from highways and traffic remained untouched. But there is nothing more wonderful at this time than the prison camp of the Muslims–may God free them!–in the Arsenal of Seville: there were thousands but the

> plague did not touch them although it practically destroyed the town itself. The report is also correct that the itinerant nomads living in tents in North Africa and elsewhere remained healthy because there the air is not shut in and the corruption proceeding from it could only gain a slight hold.

Then Ibn-al-Khaṭīb attacks the jurists who with their teaching about the non-existence of contagion were guilty of the death of countless people although they had acted in good faith by basing themselves on the external sense of the Ḥadīth *lā ʿadwā*. He continues:

> But it belongs to principles which one may not ignore that a proof taken from tradition (Ḥadīth), if observation and inspection are contrary, must be interpreted allegorically. In this matter it is essential that it should be interpreted in accordance with the views of those who hold the theory of contagion. There are numerous compassionate passages in revealed scripture, for example, the utterance of the Prophet: 'an owner of sick animals should not drive these to the owner of healthy animals.'

The special thing about these writings of 1348 is that in them for the first time the plague (caused by the bacillus *Pasteurella pestis*) is conceived as an independent illness and is separated from the confused cluster of 'epidemic' or 'pestilential illnesses', about which al-Majūsī, Pseudo-Thābit ibn-Qurra, Ibn-Sīnā and others spoke. Ibn-Khātima and Ibn-al-Khaṭīb are the first to give us exact descriptions of the symptoms which make it possible to identify the illness in its different forms as bubonic plague or pneumonic plague. Previously Ibn-al-Khaṭīb's recognition of infection was seen as his special achievement.[27] This was mistaken because Ibn-al-Khaṭīb was only repeating here what had been generally recognized from time immemorial by doctors and in the administrative practice of the towns. His suggestion, to interpret the Ḥadīth *lā ʿadwā* allegorically, was in no way revolutionary. He carried on the debate with the theologians carefully, despite invective. Besides, one must not think that Ibn-al-Khaṭīb developed his own theory about contagion as did Gerolamo Fracastoro two hundred years later in his book, *De contagionibus, et contagiosis morbis, et eorum curatione, libri tres*, Venice 1546.[28]

The Arabs published an abundance of plague literature in the centuries following the Black Death epidemic, but the sober, enlightened tone of Ibn-al-Khaṭīb is no longer heard in them. Rather, there appears increasingly in them the standpoint of a stiff-necked dogmatism. Bigotry and magic dissolve rational reflection with amulets and prayers. Such a work is, for example, the *Kitāb Badhl al-māʿūn* by Ibn-Ḥajar al-ʿAsqalānī (d. 1448), who stresses that the plague also had its good side because those who died of it were held to be martyrs.[29]

From now on there is no more room among Arabic authors for the idea of infection. It was the Europeans who reintroduced it into Arabic lands. When the plague descended on the Iberian peninsula and North Africa in 1521–2, the Portuguese governor of Arzila took all measures to shut off the town from the outside world. Three Moroccan prisoners of war who were brought into the town despite the prohibition, were compelled to bathe in the sea several times and their clothes were burnt. In vain! The plague spread in Arzila. Most of the women and children were sent back to Portugal where they spent two months in quarantine. Of those who remained behind, the plague claimed 1200 victims between January and June.[30]

SEVEN

DIETETICS AND PHARMACEUTICS

Dietetics

'The science of medicine', al-Majūsī writes,[1] 'can be divided into three parts. The first is the science of the "natural things", the second the science of the "non-natural things", the third the science of the "extra-natural things".'

By 'natural things' is meant the elements, the temperament, the humours, the faculties, the pneumata, etc., in fact, everything that is the subject of physiology, as we tried to sketch it in the fourth chapter. The 'extra-natural things' are the illnesses, their causes and their symptoms. We have spoken about these in the chapter on pathology. There remain the 'non-natural things', a vast area to which al-Majūsī dedicates the entire fifth section of the first part of his work.[2] He explains that it is about six things absolutely essential to man to preserve life: 1) the air around us; 2) movement and rest; 3) eating and drinking; 4) sleeping and waking; 5) the natural excretion and retention (to which belong also bathing and coitus) and 6) the soul's moods – joy, anger, sadness and the like. These things are not 'natural' or 'innate' in the sense that the elements, humours or pneumata are, but neither are they, as man now is, 'extra-natural' or foreign to him. If they are in fact used quantitatively and qualitatively in the right way and at the right time and in the right order, they preserve the 'natural things' in their right condition. Thus they guarantee the health of the body, until the latter succumbs to natural decay, that is, death by old age. But if these things are used other than as advised, they drive the body out of its natural condition and engender in it illnesses, and prolong these illnesses.

But these six things must be treated differently and individually. If a body, for example, has a balanced temperament, its owner should follow a balanced way of life. Spring-like air is good for him, he should indulge in exercise in moderation, bath in moderately warm water, should not sleep too little or too much, should only practise coitus when he feels happy and refreshed, when his stomach is not too full nor too empty, and when he is neither hot nor cold. In a body which deviates from the right proportion, a way of life must be followed which deviates from the right proportion in the same degree but in the opposite direction. In this way the fault will be corrected and right proportion restored. For example: if a man of fiery temperament undertakes too much physical work, he only increases the unnatural heat of his body; this injures him, weakens his faculties and produces fever. If he only undertakes a little work, this brings his innate heat into equilibrium; this promotes the health and strength of his body.

These short theoretical remarks of al-Majūsī's make it strikingly clear how greatly the medieval concepts differ from our own. Purely fictitious entities like the elements, the humours, the pneumata, are numbered among the 'natural things'; they form the physiology of man in the real sense. Breathing, eating and elimination, sleeping and waking, central physiological processes by our way of thinking, were then known as the 'non-naturals'. We shall not discuss here how this expression grew out of the ancient sphygmology;[3] sufficient to say that it is used by Ḥunayn and al-Majūsī to denote the wide field of dietetics, of right and sound living. Naturally breathing and digestion are also special physiological procedures for these medieval doctors. If they are here listed, together with movement and rest or the disciplining of the psychical moods, among the 'non-naturals', it becomes clear that the accent lies on the conscious, reasonable ruling of these processes. Man is free to form his way of life so that health and sickness are dependent on his behaviour. Compared with the instinctive way of life of the animal, these six things in man are indeed 'non-natural'.

A second thing too, becomes clear: al-Majūsī had said that when a body deviates from the right proportion, a life style must be followed which deviates from the right proportion in the same degree but in the opposite direction. The life style

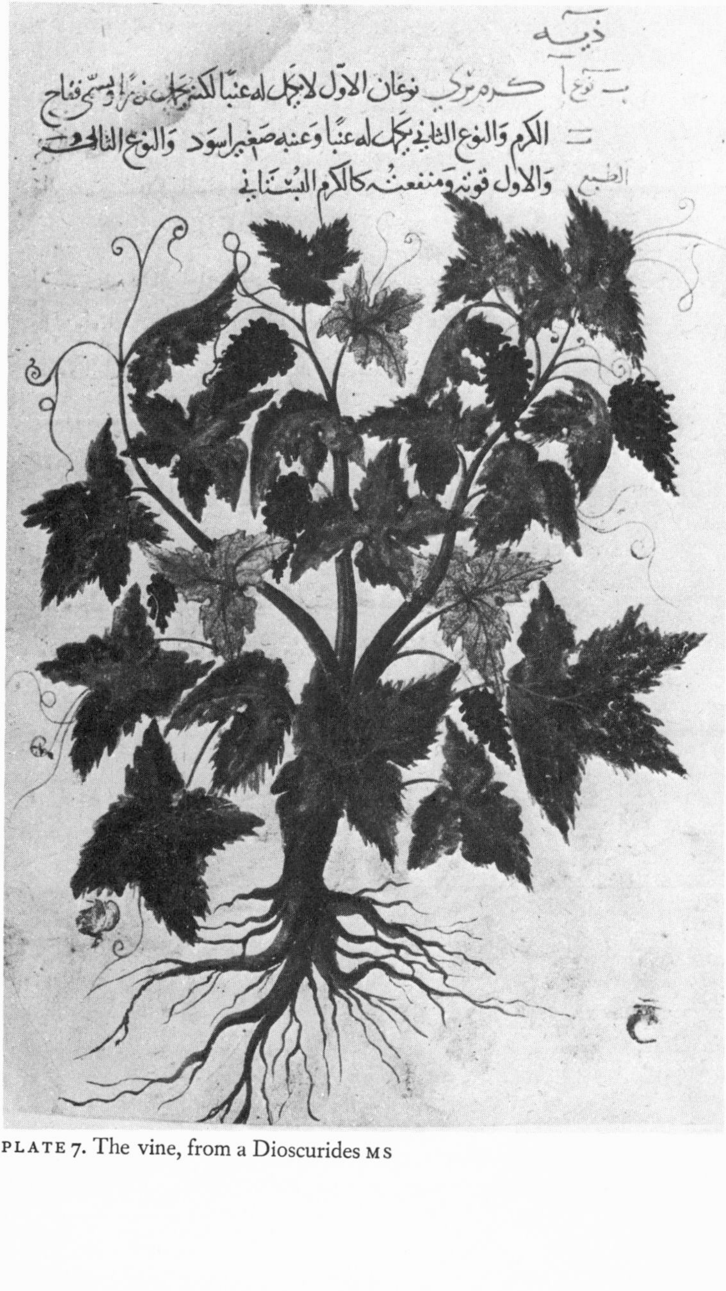

PLATE 7. The vine, from a Dioscurides MS

fruct' mandragore.

fructus mandragore. cpfo fri. mi. sic.i ?. Electo magni odouferi. vinani. odoiado ocra sed.i
caam. 7 vigilias. emplando elefanne 7 ifectoiby nigris cutis. nocumi. ebetat sensus. Re-
noeti. cu fructu edere. Quid gnat no e comestibilesjuenit ca.iuviby estate 7 midianis.

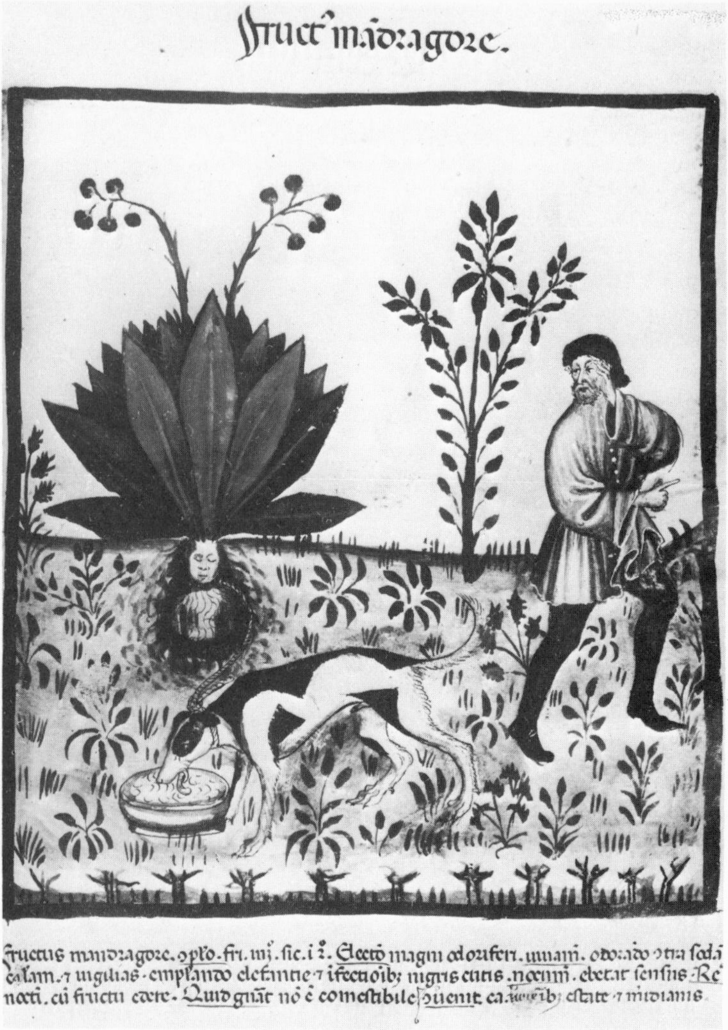

PLATE 8. Pulling out of the mandrake root, according to
the Latin *Tacuinum sanitatis in medicina*

must therefore be oriented on the principle '*contraria contrariis*'. This is a therapeutic principle, that is, dietetics become an important therapeutic means alongside surgery and pharmaceutics. In many cases the patient can be made healthy again simply by a change of life style.[4] Therefore the doctors very often prefer to prescribe suitable food because they fear the fierceness of the remedies.

The catalogue of the 'six non-naturals' follows an old tradition. These six subdivisions of vital activity are already taken into consideration in the formulary (*pinakidion*) according to which the Hippocratic doctor arranged his prescription.[5] The Arabs have produced a superfluity of books on hygiene. Works in which the whole field of hygiene is treated were published by Qusṭā ibn-Lūqā, Is'ḥāq ibn-'Imrān, Ibn-al-Jazzār, Ibn-Sīnā, Ibn-Buṭlān (*Kitāb Taqwīm aṣ-ṣiḥḥa*, in Latin *Tacuinum sanitatis*), Fakhr-ad-Dīn ar-Rāzī, al-Burqumānī, Ibn-al-Quff, Lisān-ad-Dīn ibn-al-Khaṭīb, and others. Alongside them are works intended for individual patients. Thus Ibn-al-Muṭrān and Maimonides published special *regimina sanitatis* for Saladin or Nūr-ad-Dīn, Saladin's son. Other writings deal only with sections of dietetics: Ḥunayn ibn-Is'ḥāq, Muḥammad ibn-Zakariyyā' ar-Rāzī, Is'ḥāq al-Isrā'īlī, Avenzoar, as-Samarqandī and many others, wrote about food. Finally, there is a series of shorter treatises on 'the way of life of the traveller', on the 'visit to the bath', on the 'ptisan' etc. The works too, on 'sexual intercourse' belong here; sometimes they confine themselves to recommending aphrodisiacs, sometimes they border on pornography. At any rate, the abundance of literature documents the importance given to dietetics in the world of medieval medicine.

In the following pages some characteristic points will be described from the writings of our chief source, the *Kitāb al-Malakī* of al-Majūsī.

Al-Majūsī gives a lot of space to the explanation of the 'airs' in the first section. The air, drawn in by breathing, changes our temperament: clear, pure air makes the humours and pneumata clear and pure; unclear and misty air has the opposite effect. The doctor must therefore observe the air conditions and the change of the seasons, as Hippocrates taught in his book *De aere aquis locis*. Pestilential air engenders epidemic illnesses and plague. This was treated more fully above on p. 89.

The second section of the 'non-naturals' is given over to physical activity and rest. Here al-Majūsī distinguishes in extremely dry fashion between light and heavy, partial and total, active and passive movement, between movement in the course of doing one's work and activity prescribed by the doctor, that is, exercise, taken to include boxing, running, ball games, riding, mountaineering etc. All this must be prescribed exactly and determined by the heat of the body. Bathing too, which really belongs to the chapter on elimination, is considered here, because a healthy person takes a bath after physical exercise or effort in order to evacuate the constituents of which he did not rid himself through physical movement, further, to compensate for the drying out of the body which is a result of movement, and finally, that the body may be purified from dirt. The most favourable time to visit the bath is the time after work and before eating (this presupposes that one only eats once a day, namely in the evening). If one baths after the meal, the head is filled with waste matter, the food sinks down undigested and blocks the food channels, so that in the long term dropsy may occur. It is quite different if someone has a loosely-knit body with wide pores for then he can easily rid himself of the waste matter in his body.

At the beginning of the third section, which deals with eating and drinking, al-Majūsī defines the concepts of drugs and nourishment. He distinguishes four categories: 1) remedies in the absolute sense are the materials which the body at first changes but which then change the body and transform it into their temperament; 2) deadly poisons are those materials which change the body and gain power over it without the body being able to resist them; 3) remedial food materials are those which at first change the body until the body gains power over them and transforms them into its own nature; belonging to this group are, for example, lettuce, ptisan, onions and garlic; 4) finally, the (pure) foods are those which the body changes and transforms into itself. Thus we have here a scholarly systematization of Galen's teaching, according to which the drug changes the physis of the body, while on the other hand the food increases its substance.[6] Al-Majūsī's scale ranges from 'food-stuffs' through 'remedial food-stuffs' to the 'remedies' and ends with the 'poisons'. Al-Majūsī again discusses all this in his chapter on pharmaceutics.

What follows now[7] is a scientific study of diet very finely graded and differentiated, in which he explains the dietetic characteristics, the temperaments, and the degree of effectiveness of types of cereals, of leguminous plants, vegetables, root crops, fruits, types of meat, types of milk, of honey and sweetmeats, of water, of drinks, and of aromatic herbs and perfumes. The subtility of this casuistic treatment is most clearly seen in the fact that perfumes too, are included in the rule of life. It is said of musk that it is warm and dry in the third degree, it quietens and strengthens the heart in people of cold temperament; it also strengthens the weak organs. If one sniffs it, together with saffron and camphor, it helps to prevent facial paralysis (*paralysis facialis*) and headaches which come from phlegm; it also strengthens a cold brain.

Finally, the choice of clothing material is important because it influences the body temperature. Linen clothes cool the heat economy of the body, especially when freshly washed; if they have already been worn for a time, they warm the body a little. The softer any cotton materials are, the more they warm the body; these must be worn in winter. Many fabrics have, however, direct therapeutic effects; silk is warm; it is good for the body and good for the back and kidneys.

The fourth section deals with sleeping and waking. It is a short chapter in which the following theory is put forward. Natural sleep comes when the brain is moderately wet, that is, when good, pure, moist vapours rise to the brain as a result of intake of food by the body. (Again he presupposes one meal a day in the evening.) Sleep has a double purpose; it quietens the brain, the senses and all psychical functions; the natural animal functions, for example breathing and digestion, however, continue. The second function of sleep is the digestion of food and the maturing of the humours. The 'innate heat' permeates in sleep to the depths of the body in order to digest the food and allow the humours to mature. Thus it is that in winter, when the nights and sleep last longer, digestion occurs more thoroughly. The individual must consider disciplined sleeping habits. To sleep too long debilitates the psychical faculties and cools the body; it increases phlegm and weakens the 'innate heat'. Too short a sleep weakens breathing and digestion, and dries out the body.

In the fifth section, dealing with the various types of elimination, he first deals with cohabitation. Its purpose is to preserve the species and is tied up with feelings of pleasure because most human beings and all animals strive after pleasure and not after descendants. The semen is formed in the body as a secretion but is not to be compared with other secretions, like nasal phlegm, saliva, sweat and urine, because it comes from the very best body substance, namely, from the clear, pure blood with which the cardinal organs are nourished. If an individual practises coitus to excess, his power will be weakened, his body become dessicated, and he begins to tremble. For his sexual organs, in order to form new semen, attract the blood that is really meant to nourish the cardinal organs. On the other hand, the body also suffers when the semen which has collected in the vessels is not eliminated. All other secretions must also be eliminated. If no coitus takes place, then there is pollution. But if nature is not even able to produce pollution, the hips become tense, the body becomes torpid, and in bad cases there may be fever. Sometimes the vapours that develop from the dammed-up semen, rise to the brain and bad concomitants can occur, for example, melancholy. Thus coitus is a valuable therapy for melancholics. Briefly, if coitus is wisely practised, it helps to maintain good health and can even cure some illnesses.

The case is similar with the remaining secretions and excretions, with stools, urine, menstrual blood. They damage the body when they are retained, or when they leave the body too suddenly. If an individual retains his faeces and meteorisms, he may get colic, diarrhoea, a fainting fit, anorexia, or shortness of breath. If eliminations are too severe, he becomes weak and without strength.

Finally, in the sixth section, al-Majūsī deals with the soul's moods, their influence on the body being taken for granted. They are just as capable of producing an illness as anything else and must therefore be controlled. Whoever gets angry for the slightest reason, is sad, or fearful or suspicious, may succumb to bad illnesses, and even die. Whoever, on the other hand, overcomes his temper and suppresses such moods with the power of his reason, will hardly be attacked by any illnesses.

Al-Majūsī's remarks about dietetics have been reported on at some length because in them once again, it becomes very clear that medieval Arabic medicine is a system complete in itself. All biological phenomena could be explained with sufficient exactness using the concepts of hot and cold, of blood and phlegm, of the attractive and repellent faculty. The explanations may seem to us naive, the system may appear to us too scholastic. However, these rules for living are so sensible that they could be broadly accepted by the modern reader. The ancient notion of moderation is everywhere in the background. It gave its stamp to this dietary and ensured its success over the centuries and millennia.

Pharmaceutics

In previous chapters it was shown that traditionally, therapy was broken up into three parts, namely, surgery, dietetics and pharmaceutics. The latter sphere had perhaps the greatest practical significance in medieval medicine, but in pharmaceutics too, there are again two sharply differentiated subdivisions; the use of simple and of compounded remedies. Galen had written large works on the *pharmaka haplā* and the *pharmaka syntheta*, the book *De simplicium medicamentorum temperamentis ac facultatibus* and the book *De compositione medicamentorum secundum locos et secundum genera*. This literary model determined the entire pharmaceutical literature of the Arabs, a corpus of endless extent. The Arabic bibliographers recognize more than a hundred authors who wrote about materia medica. But only a few of these works are original, independent achievements. Most are compilations and hardly in any other branch of literature has so much been copied as here. And so Albrecht von Haller is not altogether wrong when he says of the Arabic authors: 'Omnes Arabes fratres sunt fraterrimi, ut qui unum eorum de plantis legerit, legerit fere omnes.'[8]

Here, however, we are not concerned to present Arabic pharmacologists and their works. It is sufficient to say that Dioscurides was indisputably the greatest authority, that his work was many times translated and elaborated and that such important scholars as Ibn-Juljul, Ibn-al-Jazzār, Abū-r-Rayḥān al-Bīrūnī, Abū-ʿUbayd al-Bakrī, the philosopher Ibn-Bājja (Avempace), the geographer al-Idrīsī and ʿAbd-al-Laṭīf al-Baghdādī, all published books on drugs in addition to their other works. Here we want rather to discuss some propositions in the theory of simple remedies, again following al-Majūsī.[9]

He who would treat illnesses must know the powers (*quwā*), effects (*afʿāl*) and benefits (*manāfiʿ*) of simples. The powers are of three kinds: the 'primary powers' are the mixtures or temperaments of the drugs. The 'secondary powers' result from the temperaments; they encourage maturation, they soften, harden, block, open, loosen, deaden pain etc. The 'tertiary powers', for example, make the stones in the bladder crumble, drive out the urine and the menses, help to expectorate phlegm, produce semen and milk.

But how can one know that a drug has a certain temperament, a certain power and effect? Al-Majūsī therefore asks the question about 'primary powers'. There are six criteria (*qawānīn*) by which drugs can be tested. The first and surest method consists in trying them out on a sick and a healthy body. But in doing so, Galen says that eight conditions must be observed: a) the drug must be free from every accidental quality; b) the illness must be simple not complex; c) contrary illnesses must be treated with the drug; d) the drug must be more powerful than the illness so that its effect can be clearly seen; e) one must note the length of time in which contrary effects appear so that one can determine which of the two effects is only accidental; f) one must look into whether the effect of a drug is the same for everybody at every time; if this is so, the effect lies in the nature of the drug; otherwise the effect is only accidental; g) one must see if the effect of a drug is specific for human beings; in an animal it can have another effect; h) one must distinguish between foods and drugs; a drug warms the body by its quality, a food by its entire substance.

The second method consists of examining whether a drug can be transformed quickly or with difficulty. This gives information about the heat of its temperament. If it is brought near fire and it quickly goes up in flames, it is potentially hot.

By the third method, observing how quickly or slowly a drug melts and congeals, one gets information about the cold of its temperament. If one takes two drugs whose substance is equally coarse or fine, the one that hardens more quickly is the colder.

The fourth method consists of examining a drug by its taste. There are eight qualities of taste: the sweet, the fatty, the acid, the bitter, the pungent (*ḥirrīf*), the salty, the bilious, and the astringent. All that is sweet is of equal heat. Because of this it produces torpor and maturation, without overheating. Everything bitter is earth-like. Therefore it cleans the vessels, it opens obstructions, and warms a little. Everything that is bilious or astringent is cold and earthlike. Consequently it thickens the pores and cools.

The fifth method, judging drugs by their smell, is not so reliable as the previous method; on the one hand, there are many things that give off no smell, on the other hand, there are things that are composed of different elements. The rose, for example, smells nice, but its taste is sometimes bitter, sometimes bilious, sometimes watery. It is not homoeomeral (*ghayr mutashābih al-ajzā'*), but has different powers: the bitter in it is hot and fine, the bilious is coarse and cold, the watery is insipid in taste and is intermediate between coarseness and fineness.

Finally, there is the sixth method which is to judge a drug by its colour. It is not of much value because with every colour there can be a hot, cold, wet or dry temperament. The most one can say is that a certain drug is less hot if it is white, that on the other hand it has more heat if it is red or black. Here the intensity of the quality depends on the degree of ripeness of the fruit or the seed.

One acquires knowledge about the 'secondary powers' of the drug if one knows the measure of the temperament of every single drug. The temperament of the 'burning' drugs has the highest degree of heat and their substance is coarse. If they are applied to the body, thanks to the force of its heat, they quickly penetrate the body and they remain in it because they are coarse. One can see this in cauterization. Drugs which allow wounds to scab and heal are the ones which firm and dry the flesh, and make it into something like skin. These drugs must accordingly be astringent and, in moderation, drying.

We do not learn much from al-Majūsī about the 'tertiary powers'. It is only stated that the drugs exercise these powers through the secondary powers by means of the temperament.

Instead of a definition he gives examples: drugs that crumble stones in the bladder are hot and stop the coarse humours; the heat must however be slight because very hot and drying methods are precisely those that allow stones to develop. So one takes the roots of asparagus, peony, etc.

This is essentially Galen's theory. Galen insists that the 'primary' powers or qualities (he uses the expressions *dynameis* and *poiotētes* interchangeably) can be deduced from the perceptions of the senses. But the decisive thing when judging a remedy is its effect upon a person. Galen too, speaks of 'secondary' and 'tertiary' powers, but the latter play a subordinate role. These are effects which come about when a drug is applied and produces certain bodily reactions.

It is striking that al-Majūsī occasionally gives the degree of effect of a drug but that he does not theoretically establish such grading. This agrees with Galen's procedure; his teaching about degrees or grades, according to most recent research, does not amount to more than a few remarks.[10] In the long list of simples with which al-Majūsī follows the introductory chapters, the details of degree are often missing. We can be sure that he had not once tested what Galen says about the powers and therapeutic effects of individual drugs. But we may also doubt whether the Arabs subjected the many new drugs of oriental and Indian origin, not yet known to the Greeks, to an examination according to Galenic criteria. Presumably they relied on what the experiences of Indian doctors or folklore ascribed to these drugs. Thus the Galenic criteria remained, broadly speaking, lifeless theory for the Arabs. They took them over from the ancients and handed them on, but like so much of their medicine, they were mere book knowledge.

EIGHT

MEDICINE AND THE OCCULT

In the first chapter, pre-Islamic medicine was described as a folk-medicine strongly influenced by magical elements. The Hellenization of Islam had confronted this folk-medicine with a highly sophisticated system of scientific medicine from which magic was banned.[1] The enlightened tendency had already begun in the *Corpus hippocraticum*. In the work *De sacro morbo*, epilepsy was given a place in the phenomenal world explained by cause and effect, and the same rationalism was found in Galen. But under the Roman empire and especially in late antiquity, a change of direction made itself felt. Magical remedies play a large role in Alexander of Tralles and he calls them *physika*, 'natural remedies'. This will seem paradoxical to us but can be explained by another concept of nature. Alexander, like Arnald of Villanova and Paracelsus at a later date, believed that the ultimate secrets of the natural faculties and the effects of medicine are concealed from us and that therefore popular and magical remedies, however inexplicable these may be, cannot just be neglected.[2] It is unimportant that these remedies seem to us absurd, disgusting and unhygienic. For Alexander they were just as 'scientifically established' as the remedies recommended by Dioscurides and Galen, and actually for him there were no criteria by which to distinguish 'natural' and 'magical' remedies. The turning towards magic therefore was not born of sheer superstition and the desire for miracles, but is almost necessarily the result of the boundaries which were set to medieval man's desire for knowledge. He scarcely knew anything about experiment which could have made possible the verification or falsification of traditional data, and mistakes in therapy which were unavoidable, were unable to shake his belief in magical lore since the postulate meant more to him than the actual experience.

Many Arabic doctors, too, adopted this attitude. In one of the earliest works of Arabic medicine, the *Paradise of Wisdom* by ʿAlī ibn-Sahl aṭ-Ṭabarī (completed in 850), much space is devoted to the presentation of sympathetic effects and magical remedies. Many miraculous things were reported on the authority of the *Physiologus*, of the *Cyranis*, of Dioscurides, of Alexander, or of authors of 'organo-therapy', like Xenocrates of Aphrodisias. ʿAlī says for example: 'If you put a magnetic stone into the hand of a woman in labour, it will help her in a difficult birth.' In another passage we read: 'I once saw a small stone that was beneficial against smallpox which resembled a mussel shot through with red', or: 'I once saw an Indian stone tied to the stomach of a dropsy sufferer and drawing the water out of him.' Other examples read: 'If a woman eats the flesh of a swallow when her period is finished, she will not become pregnant for a whole year.' 'If the heart of the wall gecko is hung round a woman, it prevents abortion.' 'The wall gecko, caught and wrapped up alive in a cloth and hung round someone suffering from intermittent fever, removes the fever.' 'If a woman was once pregnant but is no longer so, she should take a frog from the river, spit in its mouth, and throw it back into the river. When her husband has intercourse with her, she will become pregnant, with God's permission.'

Similarly, ʿAlī recounts many practices carried out in his Persian homeland, especially in Tabaristan. 'The director of the hospital in Gondēshāpūr told me about a family in al-Ahwāz who possess a stone which protects the foetus if hung round the pregnant woman. If by chance she meets another pregnant woman, the latter, who possesses no stone, aborts.' Another account runs: 'In the mountains of Tabaristan, the panther often beats a man with his paw. Then mice gather round him from all sides and the men and women must ensure that the mice do not reach him, since if they urinate on him, he must die.' Furthermore we read: 'The people of Tabaristan say that if one lights a fire from the wood of a fig tree in front of a man suffering from a hydrocele, his testicles will return to their normal place.'

Next to ʿAlī ibn-Sahl, it is the famous doctor Muḥammad ibn-Zakariyyā' ar-Rāzī, well-known for his sober clinical observations, who believed in the existence of occult powers. Indeed, he wrote a book, the *Kitāb al-Khawāṣṣ*, specifically on this subject. And in his book *Kitāb al-Ḥāwī*, he frequently recommends magical remedies and occasionally also quotes Balīnās (i.e. Apollonius of Tyana) and his book *Kitāb aṭ-Ṭabī-ʿiyyāt* (= *Physika*), as well as a similar work by Hermes. Ar-Rāzī teaches, following this source, that quartan fever can be cured if the patient wears the unwashed and sweaty shirt of a woman in labour (in this case sweat and the difference of sex are alike effective in transmitting power).[3] His book goes on: 'If one eats a scorpion, it will break up the stones in the bladder, and if one eats earth worms after one has squashed them, they will break up the stones in the bladder.'[4] 'If the hair of a woman is burnt and applied to a bleeding part, it will stop the bleeding completely.'[5] He recommends the following for scorpion stings: 'If you squash a scorpion and lay it on the wound, this will help considerably.'[6]

Sympathetic remedies are especially practised in midwifery. Characteristic of this is a chapter in the large work on pregnancy and the care of infants (*Kitāb al-Ḥabālā wa-l-aṭfāl*) written by Aḥmad ibn-Muḥammad al-Baladī, a doctor who served as physician to the Egyptian vizier Abū-l-Faraj Yaʿqūb ibn-Yūsuf ibn-Killis in the tenth century.[7] There, among other things, al-Baladī gives the following instructions to ease birth: 'If one wraps an onyx in the hair of the woman in labour, she will produce the child immediately. Even if it is placed near her, it will drive away all pains.' 'A snake-skin wound around the hips of the woman, accelerates the birth.' 'If you pull up the coriander carefully and hang the root fibres over the thigh of the woman, it will help the birth.'

This last example shows clearly that care is advocated even when collecting a drug. Occasionally too, the time and the position of the stars must be taken into account when collecting medicinal plants, sometimes to the extent of carrying out complicated ceremonies. According to Hermes,[8] the root of the mandrake or alruna which has the form of an idol with all human limbs, gives protection not only against all mental illness, like madness, forgetfulness, melancholy, but also against apoplexy, elephantiasis etc. If one is going to pull the root out of the earth, it must be done at the right time. Mars must be in one of his houses, preferably in the highest house, Aries, or in the house of his exaltation (*sharaf*), Capricorn. If Venus and Jupiter stand in a favourable aspect to him, so much the better. The moon must be in conjunction with Mars or be together with him in his zodiacal sign. If these conditions are complied with, one can set about the uprooting at dawn on Tuesday. The advocates of these esoteric actions claim that one can only pull up the mandrake root if the earth round about has been loosened. The mandrake must be tied to the neck of a dog which has been starved for a day. When one calls the dog to one from some distance, the dog in the course of running pulls up the root but drops dead to the ground.[9]

Arabic pharmaceutical literature is full of such and similar instructions and it is stones that are most popularly used in magical cures. A glance in a round mirror of polished jet protects against cataract, writes at-Tamīmī in his *Kitāb al-Murshid*.[10]

A whole genre of literature was devoted to magic. These are the *Kutub al-Mujarrabāt* and there are more than a dozen authors who are supposed to have written such '*empirica*'. The prescriptions in these books are supposed to be 'confirmed by experience' but this is only propaganda or self-deception, since they are really dealing with remedies whose effects are outwith experience. It is pure magic as one of a thousand examples shows: 'If one burns the bones of the sand grouse and boils up the ashes from these with the oil made from unripe olives and with this rubs the head of a bald person and the patches of alopecia, the hair will grow again. Tried (*mujarrab*).' The characteristic word *mujarrab* at the end of this prescription is the same as the note frequently written on Alexander of Tralles's prescriptions: *pepeiratai*.[11]

The stronger inclination towards magic can perhaps be partly explained by the fact that ancient oriental magical practices which had continued underground in the hellenized countries, had flooded into Greek literature from imperial times and had conquered a wide field. At least in one case the path to the Arabs from ancient oriental medicine via late Hellenistic literature can be followed exactly: this is the *Cyranis*, a treatise, which, as we are informed, originated in Babylon. In it plants, birds, stones and fish, are grouped alphabetically, and each of these creatures either individually or in combination can be used in magical rites and cures. In *Cyranis*, Alpha 37, we read: 'If the stone from the head of the "eagle fish" is hung round the neck of a sufferer from quartan fever, the patient will be cured', and the instruction in Omega 32 runs: 'On the stone found in the head of the Ōmis-fish one should engrave a swallow superimposed on the picture of a scorpion and should draw the picture of this fish looking towards the picture of the scorpion, and take the eyes of the scorpion and the fish, as well as part of the root of the "scorpion-tree" and bring this under the ring-stone before fixing it (to the ring). Whoever wears this signet-ring is safe from all vermin on earth. Even though an animal bites him, this will not hurt him.' The *Cyranis* was translated from Syriac(?) into Greek in the second or third century A.D. and further translated from Greek into Arabic, thus finding its way back again to the East.[12] But as we have seen, old Iranian magical ideas were directly transmitted by ʿAlī ibn-Sahl to the Arabs.

Medicine and astrology

The attitude of Islamic doctors to astrology was just as varied as their relationship to magic. Many doctors were also astrologers, for example, Yaḥyā ibn-Jarīr at-Takrītī (*c.* 1030) or ʿAlī ibn-Riḍwān (d. 1068) who made a name for himself with his commentary on the *Quadripartitum* of Ptolemy. The philosopher Yaʿqūb ibn-Is'ḥāq al-Kindī, who also published several medical works, wrote a treatise *De signis astronomiae applicatis ad medicinam* which is only preserved in the Latin translation. In a further writing, the *Risāla fī ʿIllat al-baḥārīn li-l-amrāḍ al-ḥādda*, al-Kindī gives astrological and iatromathematical reasons for the periodicity of the crises.[13]

Again and again in vindication of the astrological tendencies we find the word quoted from the Hippocratic writing *De aere aquis locis* which tells how 'the science of the stars (*astronomiē*) performs no small service to medical science, indeed an extremely large one'. In the context of this writing are meant chiefly the rising and setting of individual constellations by means of which the doctor can determine the beginning and end of the seasons. The text continues: 'For sometimes a change in the bodily cavity of men coincides with the change in the seasons'. But the doctors interested in astrology took the first sentence out of its context and used it in their own way. Thus ʿAlī ibn-Sahl aṭ-Ṭabarī in his *Paradise of Wisdom*, following on what Hippocrates had said, gives a full presentation of the basic concepts of astrology and astronomy and even Muḥammad ibn-Zakariyyā' ar-Rāzī in his *Kitāb al-Ḥāwī* has a short section on the influence of the stars on the crises of illnesses.[14]

In several works the question is dealt with as to what astrological knowledge is necessary for doctors. Typical of this is the *Risāla fī-mā yaḥtāj aṭ-ṭabīb min ʿilm al-falak* by Abū-Naṣr ʿAdnān ibn-Naṣr al-ʿAynzarbī (d. 1153), personal physician to the Fatimid caliph aẓ-Ẓāfir bi-Amr-Allāh in Cairo. After he had by way of introduction referred to the saying of Hippocrates already mentioned, he explained that the individual planets in certain positions prognosticate certain illnesses. The doctor must utilize the knowledge of these things for diagnostic and prognostic purposes. Especially in the case of bleeding, the stellar constellations must be observed. For example, we read: 'Bleeding of the neck is unfavourable if the moon is in the sign of Taurus, that of the back when the moon is in the sign of Leo . . . and generally, when the moon is in the sign of that limb which is to be cupped.' Such rules about cupping were popularly acknowledged. In the *Arabian Nights* we read: 'When your father said to me, "draw my blood", I fetched the astrolabe and found that the constellation of the hour was unfavourable'.[15] Consultations with astrologers were part and parcel of life generally: when the sultan al-Malik an-Nāṣir Muḥammad ibn-Qalāwūn became ill with diarrhoea, not only the doctors but also the astrologers and geomancers were asked for their opinion.[16]

Often the development of the foetus in the womb is represented from an astrological standpoint. ʿArīb ibn-Saʿīd of Cordova (d. *c.* 980)[17] recounts the following sequence of development in his *Kitāb Khalq al-janīn wa-tadbīr al-ḥabālā wa-l-mawlūdīn*:

> In the first month, when the foetus is still a formless drop, it stands under the sway of Saturn, whose nature is cold and dry. Because of this, the drop has no sense perception and no movement. In the second month it stands under

the sway of Jupiter, whose nature is hot and wet. Now it begins to grow and to form into a lump of flesh. If it is a boy, its colour is white and its shape round: if it is a girl, its colour is red and its shape like that of a banana. In the third month Mars, who is hot and dry, holds sway. At this stage nerves and blood appear in the lump of flesh. The sun, which is likewise hot and dry, determines the fourth month when the foetus begins to move. When in the fifth month cold Venus holds sway, the brain, the bones and the skin form. Mercury, relatively hot and dry, influences development in the sixth month, when the tongue and the hearing develop. In the seventh month the foetus stands under the sway of the moon whose attributes are swift movements. By now the child is fully formed and thrusts outwards. If it is actually born this month, it can live, and grow, because it has experienced the influences of the seven planets in their entirety. However, if it remains in the womb, it again comes under the sway of Saturn in the eighth month, which is cold and dry. This quietens it, even makes it ill, so that if born now, it cannot live. But in the ninth month, Jupiter rules again, bringer of life and growth. If the child is born now, it will live and the same applies to the tenth month.[18]

A very similar sequence of development is given by al-Majūsī[19] who wants to explain why an eight-month-old child is incapable of life. Strangely enough, he believes this astrological thesis justified by the explanation given by Hippocrates in his book *De octimestri partu*. According to Hippocrates, the child goes through a process of transformation in the eighth month which weakens it, and if born then, it cannot live.

Interesting is the division and characterization of the different ages of life which we will report according to ʿArīb ibn-Saʿīd. ʿArīb says that according to the astrologers, the first four years of a child's life are determined by the cold and wet moon whose sphere is nearest to our earth. For this reason, the small child is weak, fragile, stupid, and can only eat a little. These four years correspond to the four elements. The following ten years form the second period of life under the dominance of Mercury, whose sphere lies over that of the moon. During this period, the child shows signs of attention, reflection and the power of discrimination, so that he can take the first steps in the sciences. Childhood ends at the age of fourteen. Venus, the next higher planet, rules over the following eight years into which fall puberty and the desire for sexual intercourse, and in which the young person has to learn self-control. Now follow, as the fourth period of life, nineteen years under the dominance of the sun, a period of time which lasts from the age of twenty-two to forty-one. Here ambition, desire for fame and a serious attitude to life make themselves felt. It is the middle of life, just as the sun occupies a middle place between the subsolar and transsolar planets. In the fifth period of life, which lasts fifteen years until the completion of the fifty-sixth year, Mars reigns. The individual strives after earthly goods, and worries, and works. The following twelve years, that is, the period from the fifty-sixth to the sixty-eighth year of life belong to Jupiter. Now age begins to make itself felt, the individual stands back from his earthly striving and thinks about ethical values and life after death. The seventh period of life, lasting thirty years until the completion of the ninety-eighth year of life, again stands under the dominance of Saturn, which revolves in the highest sphere. The individual loses his strength, his freshness, his hope, his desires, he becomes ill and decrepit, his body becomes cold. If he survives this age, he again comes under the moon's influence and is again childish like a child.[20]

However, by and large, astrological considerations play only a small part in Arabic medicine. Whereas in the West, unfavourable conjunctions of the planets were constantly considered to be one of the chief causes of plague, Lisān-ad-Dīn ibn-al-Khaṭīb takes a conjunction of the planets to be 'a more distant cause' of the appearance of plague.[21] Avicenna himself published a book refuting astrology,[22] and his attitude is shared by the majority of the great doctors of the Islamic classical period.

ABBREVIATIONS

Browne, *Medicine* = Edward Granville Browne, *Arabian Medicine*, Cambridge 1921.
Bull. Hist. Med. = *Bulletin of the History of Medicine*, Baltimore.
CMG = *Corpus Medicorum Graecorum*, ediderunt Academiae Berolinensis, Havniensis, Lipsiensis.
Diepgen, *Medizin* = Paul Diepgen, *Geschichte der Medizin: Die historische Entwicklung der Heilkunde und des ärztlichen Lebens*, I, Berlin 1949.
Edelstein, *Ancient Medicine* = *Ancient Medicine: Selected Papers of Ludwig Edelstein*, Edited by Owsei Temkin and C. Lilian Temkin, Baltimore 1967.
*EI*² = *The Encyclopaedia of Islam* (new edition), Leiden–London 1960.
Flashar, *Antike Medizin* = *Antike Medizin*, herausgegeben von Hellmut Flashar (Wege der Forschung Bd. CCXXI) Darmstadt 1971.
Flashar, *Melancholie* = Hellmut Flashar, *Melancholie und Melancholiker in den medizinischen Theorien der Antike*, Berlin 1966.
Grabner, *Volksmedizin* = *Volksmedizin: Probleme und Forschungsgeschichte*, herausgegeben von Elfriede Grabner (Wege der Forschung Bd. LXIII) Darmstadt 1967.
Haeser, *Lehrbuch* = Heinrich Haeser, *Lehrbuch der Geschichte der Medicin und der epidemischen Krankheiten*, Dritte Bearbeitung, Bd. I-III, Jena 1875–82.
Hovorka-Kronfeld = Oskar von Hovorka und Adolf Kronfeld, *Vergleichende Volksmedizin*, Bd. I. II, Stuttgart 1908–9.
Ibn-an-Nadīm, *Fihrist* = *Kitâb al-Fihrist*, mit Anmerkungen herausgegeben von Gustav Flügel, Bd. I-II, Leipzig 1871–2.
Ibn-Sīnā, *Qānūn* = *K. al-Qānūn fī ṭ-ṭibb li-Abī-ʿAlī ibn-Sīnā*, vol. I. II, Rome 1593.
Majūsī, *Malakī* = *Al-Kitāb al-Malakī* (*K. Kāmil aṣ-ṣināʿa aṭ-ṭibbiyya*) *li-ʿAlī ibn-al-ʿAbbās al-Majūsī*, vol. I. II, Būlāq 1294.

Med. hist. J. = *Medizinhistorisches Journal*, Hildesheim.

Rāzī, *Ḥāwī* = *Kitāb al-Ḥāwī li-Muḥammad ibn-Zakariyyā' ar-Rāzī*, vol. I-XXIII, Hyderabad 1955–71.

RE = *Paulys Realencyclopädie der classischen Altertumswissenschaft*, neue Bearbeitung herausgegeben von Georg Wissowa, Stuttgart 1893ff.

Siegel, *Galen's Physiology* = Rudolph E. Siegel, *Galen's System of Physiology and Medicine: an Analysis of his Doctrines and Observations on Bloodflow, Respiration, Humors and Internal Diseases*, Basel – New York 1968.

Temkin, *Galenism* = Owsei Temkin, *Galenism: Rise and Decline of a Medical Philosophy*, Ithaca and London 1973.

Ullmann, *Medizin* = Manfred Ullmann, *Die Medizin im Islam* (Handbuch der Orientalistik, hsgb. von Bertold Spuler, Erste Abteilung, Ergänzungsband VI, 1. Abschnitt) Leiden – Köln 1970.

WKAS = *Wörterbuch der Klassischen Arabischen Sprache.* Begründet von Jörg Kraemer und Helmut Gätje. In Verbindung mit Anton Spitaler bearbeitet von Manfred Ullmann, Wiesbaden 1970.

NOTES

Introduction

1. Francesco Gabrieli, *Antaios*, IX (1968) 517.
2. Browne, *Medicine*, 113.
3. Edward Granville Browne, *Arabian Medicine*, Cambridge 1921, rep. London 1962; French translation by H. P. J. Renaud, Paris 1933.
4. Manfred Ullmann, *Die Medizin im Islam* (Handbuch der Orientalistik, hsgb. von Bertold Spuler, Erste Abteilung, Ergänzungsband VI, 1. Abschnitt) Leiden – Köln 1970.
5. Published May 1971. The title-page bears the date 1970.
6. cf. the critical review by Martin Plessner, *Ambix*, XIX (1972) 209-15.

Chapter One

1. Charles M. Doughty, *Travels in Arabia Deserta*, vol. I. II, Cambridge 1888, index s.vv. Maladies, Cauterizing, etc.
2. George A. Lipsky, *Saudi Arabia, its people, its society, its culture*, New Haven 1959, 262-76.
3. Shihāb ad-Dīn al-Khafājī, *Sharḥ Durrat al-ghawwāṣ*, Constantinople 1299, 214.
4. Heinrich Vorwahl, in: Grabner, *Volksmedizin*, 254.
5. Maxime Rodinson, *EI*², IV, 327-33 (s.v. Kabid).
6. Fridolf Kudlien, '"Schwärzliche" Organe im frühgriechischen Denken', *Med. hist. J.*, VIII (1973) 53-8.
7. Abu-ʿUbayd al-Bakrī, *Simṭ*, I, 141, 1 ff.
8. *WKAS*, I, 75 b 25 ff.; 550 b 35 ff.
9. Wolfdietrich Fischer, *Farb- und Formbezeichnungen in der Sprache der altarabischen Dichtung*, Wiesbaden 1965, 420-5.
10. Al-Huṭay'a, VIII, 18 (ed. Goldziher).
11. *WKAS*, II, 244 a 43 ff.
12. *Travels in Arabia Deserta*, vol. I, 492.
13. *WKAS*, I, 477 b 36 ff.
14. Labīd, XIV, 31 (ed. Iḥsān ʿAbbās).

15. *Mufaḍḍaliyyāt*, XV, 24f., trs. Charles Lyall.
16. Hovorka-Kronfeld, I, 79-88 (s.v. Blut); II, 431.
17. Doughty, *Travels*, vol. I, 255.
18. *Dīwān al-Hudhaliyyīn*, II, 3 (ed. Kosegarten).
19. For the medico-magical ideas of the ancient Arabs see the following sources: Ḥamza ibn-al-Ḥasan al-Iṣbahānī, *K. ad-Durra al-fākhira*, vol. II, ed. ʿAbd-al-Majīd Qaṭāmish (Dhakhā'ir al-ʿarab, 46) Cairo 1972, 552-65 (cf. Eugen Mittwoch, 'Abergläubische Vorstellungen und Bräuche der alten Araber nach Ḥamza al-Iṣbahānī' [*Mitteilungen des Seminars für Orientalische Sprachen*, XVI (1913) Abt. II: Westasiatische Studien] Berlin 1913, 1-14); Ibn-abī-l-Ḥadīd, *Sharḥ Nahj al-balāgha*, XIX, 382-429; Nuwairī, *Nihāya*, III, 116-27; Julius Wellhausen, *Reste arabischen Heidentums*, gesammelt und erläutert, 2. Ausgabe, Berlin and Leipzig 1897, 161ff.
20. *WKAS*, II, 178b9ff.
21. Wellhausen, *Reste*, 159-67; Hovorka-Kronfeld, I, 32f. (s.v. Anspucken); Rudolf Sellheim, *Oriens*, XVIII/XIX (1967) 63f. For the whole subject see Arent Jan Wensinck, *A Handbook of Early Muhammadan Tradition*, Leiden 1927, (s.vv. Medicine, Sick, Sickness, Incantation).
22. Ibn Khaldûn, *The Muqaddimah. An Introduction to History*, translated from the Arabic by Franz Rosenthal, vol. III, 2nd ed., Princeton 1967, 150.
23. Ibn-Qutayba, *Kitāb al-Maʿārif*, ed. Tharwat ʿUkkāsha, Cairo 1960, 222.
24. *Kitāb al-Aghānī*, ed. al-Bijāwī, XVII, Cairo 1970, 241.
25. Meir J. Kister, 'On the Papyrus of Wahb b. Munabbih', *Bulletin of the School of Oriental and African Studies*, XXXVII (1974) 545-71.
26. *The Natural History Section from a 9th Century 'Book of Useful Knowledge', The ʿUyûn al-Akhbâr of Ibn Qutayba*, trs. Lothar Kopf, ed. Friedrich S. Bodenheimer, Paris – Leiden 1949, 33f.
27. *The Naḳā'iḍ of Jarīr and al-Farazdaḳ*, ed. Anthony Ashley Bevan, Leiden 1905–7, nr. LXI, 23.
28. Albert Dietrich, *EI*², III, 39-43.
29. Al-Marzubānī, *K. Nūr al-qabas*, ed. R. Sellheim, Wiesbaden 1964, 49f.

Chapter Two

1. Dominique Sourdel, *EI*², I, 1141.
2. Manfred Ullmann, *Die Welt des Islams*, N.S. XIII (1971) 204–211; id., *Der Islam*, L (1973) 232f.
3. Temkin, *Galenism*, 59ff.

4. Ibn-an-Nadīm, *Fihrist*, 293f.
5. Manfred Ullmann, 'Die arabische Überlieferung der hippokratischen Schrift "De superfetatione"', *Sudhoffs Archiv*, LVIII (1974) 254-75.
6. Aḥmad ibn-abī-Ya'qūb ibn-Ja'far ibn-Wāḍiḥ, *K.at-Ta'rīkh*, ed. M. Th. Houtsma, Leiden 1883, Pars I, 107-16. I owe this information to Dr Hans Hinrich Biesterfeldt.
7. Kurt Weitzmann, 'The Greek Sources of Islamic Scientific Illustrations', *Archaeologica Orientalia in Memoriam Ernst Herzfeld*, New York 1952, 250-7.
8. *Al-Biruni's Book on Pharmacy and Materia Medica*, edited with English translation by Hakim Mohammed Said, Karachi 1973.
9. Haeser, *Lehrbuch*, I, 389f.
10. Majūsī, *Malakī*, II, 454-516 (Maqāla IX).
11. Temkin, *Galenism*, 62.
12. Ludwig Edelstein, 'Greek Medicine in its Relation to Religion and Magic', *Bulletin of the Institute of the History of Medicine*, V (1937) 201-46, reprinted in: Edelstein, *Ancient Medicine*, 205-46.
13. Manfred Ullmann, 'Die arabische Überlieferung der Kyranis des Hermes Trismegistos', *Proceedings of the VIth Congress of Arabic and Islamic Studies* [Visby–Stockholm 1972] Stockholm–Leiden 1975, 196-200.
14. Manfred Ullmann, 'Das Steinbuch des Xenokrates von Ephesos', *Med. hist. J.*, VII (1972) 49-64; id., 'Neues zum Steinbuch des Xenokrates', ibid., VIII (1973) 59-76; id., Art. 'Xenokrates', *RE*, Suppl.bd. XIV (1974) col. 974-7.
15. Fridolf Kudlien, 'Herophilos und der Beginn der medizinischen Skepsis', *Gesnerus*, XXI (1964) 1-13, reprinted in: Flashar, *Antike Medizin*, 280-95.
16. Max Wellmann, *Die pneumatische Schule bis auf Archigenes in ihrer Entwickelung dargestellt*, Berlin 1895, 24; Fridolf Kudlien, *Untersuchungen zu Aretaios von Kappadokien* (Akademie der Wissenschaften und der Literatur, Abhandl. d. geistes- und sozialwiss. Klasse, 1963, nr. 11), Wiesbaden 1964; Karl Deichgräber, *Aretaeus von Kappadozien als medizinischer Schriftsteller* (Abhandlungen der Sächsischen Akademie der Wissenschaften zu Leipzig, phil.-hist. Klasse, Bd. 63, Heft 3) Berlin 1971.
17. Manfred Ullmann, 'Yūḥannā ibn Sarābiyūn. Untersuchungen zur Überlieferungsgeschichte seiner Werke', *Med. hist. J.*, VI (1971) 278-96; Rainer Degen, 'Ein Corpus Medicorum Syriacorum', ibid., VII (1972) 114-22.
18. Henry E. Sigerist, *A History of Medicine*, vol. I, New York 1951, 356f.
19. Harold Walter Bailey, *Zoroastrian Problems in the Ninth-*

Century Books. Ratanbai Katrak Lectures, Oxford 1943, 2nd printing 1971, 81. The whole chapter 'Martōm' (pp. 78-119) shows the influence of Aristotelian and Greek medical conceptions upon the Persian anthropology of that time.

20. Arthur Christensen, *L'Iran sous les Sassanides*, deuxième édition revue et augmentée, Copenhagen 1944, 415-29.
21. cf. the excellent study by Richard Ettinghausen, *From Byzantium to Sasanian Iran and the Islamic World. Three modes of artistic influence* (The L.A. Mayer Memorial Studies in Islamic Art and Archaeology, vol. III) Leiden 1972.
22. Carlo Alfonso Nallino, 'Tracce di opere greche giunte agli Arabi per trafila Pehlevica', *A Volume of Oriental Studies presented to Edward Granville Browne*, Cambridge 1922, 345-63.
23. Paul Kunitzsch, *Der Almagest. Die Syntaxis Mathematica des Claudius Ptolemäus in arabisch-lateinischer Überlieferung*, Wiesbaden 1974, 123-5.
24. Manfred Ullmann, 'Die Schrift des Badīgūras über die Ersatzdrogen', *Der Islam*, L (1973) 230-48.
25. Ullmann, *Medizin*, 107.
26. Rāzī, *Ḥāwī*, I, 112; 258; II, 80; III, 228; VI, 134; 150; 190; 253; VIII, 58; 156; IX, 69; 147; X, 198; XI, 64; XIX, 440; XX, 445; 451; 518; XXI, 66; 147; 287; 367; 571; 590; XXIII, 1, 218.
27. Max Höfler, *Die volksmedizinische Organotherapie und ihr Verhältnis zum Kultopfer*, Stuttgart-Berlin-Leipzig, n.d.
28. Rāzī, *Ḥāwī*, III, 51.
29. Ibn-al-ʿAwwām, *Filāḥa*, II, 467.
30. Arthur Christensen, *L'Iran sous les Sassanides*, 2nd ed., Copenhagen 1944, 423 ff.; Alexander M. Honeyman, *The Mission of Burzoe in the Arabic Kalilah and Dimnah*, Chicago 1936.
31. Hermann Diels, *Die Handschriften der antiken Ärzte*, vol. II, Berlin 1906, 81.
32. Moritz Winternitz, *Geschichte der indischen Literatur*, III, Leipzig 1922, 545-7.
33. Werner Schmucker, 'Ein Beitrag zur Indo-Arabischen Arzneimittelkunde und Geistesgeschichte', *Zeitschrift der deutschen morgenländischen Gesellschaft*, CXXV (1975) 66-98.
34. Alfred Siggel, *Die indischen Bücher aus dem Paradies der Weisheit über die Medizin des ʿAlī ibn Sahl Rabban aṭ-Ṭabarī, übersetzt und erläutert* (Akademie der Wissenschaften und der Literatur, Abhandl. d. geistes- u. sozialwiss. Klasse, 1950, nr. 14) Wiesbaden 1951.
35. Ludwig Edelstein, *Bull. Hist. Med.*, VIII (1940) 759.
36. Cajus Fabricius, 'Galens Exzerpte aus älteren Pharmakologen' (*Ars Medica*, II, 2) Berlin 1972.

37. Majūsī, *Malakī*, I, 16 ult. ff.
38. ibid., 44, 27 ff.
39. ibid., 150, 31 ff.
40. *Med. hist. J.*, X (1975) 181-3.
41. W. Montgomery Watt, *The Influence of Islam on Medieval Europe* (Islamic Surveys 9) Edinburgh 1972, 30.
42. Ed. Maximilianus Wellmann, *CMG*, X, I, I, Leipzig and Berlin 1908.
43. Ullmann, *Medizin*, 334-41.
44. *Materia medica*, V, nr. 151-60.
45. Galen, *De simpl. med.*, IX, I (vol. XII, 165-92 Kühn).
46. Ibn-Sīnā, *Qānūn*, I, 184f.
47. Vol. III, 106-12.
48. Berthold Laufer, *Geophagy* (Field Museum of Natural History Publication 280, Anthropological Series vol. XVIII, No. 2) Chicago 1930, 150-5: 164-6.
49. Heinz Grotzfeld, *Das Bad im arabisch-islamischen Mittelalter. Eine kulturgeschichtliche Studie*, Wiesbaden 1970.
50. Owsei Temkin, *The Falling Sickness. A History of Epilepsy from the Greeks to the Beginnings of Modern Neurology*, 2nd ed., Baltimore and London 1971, 5, 151; *WKAS*, I, 418b25 ff.; 579b30 ff.
51. *WKAS*, I, 300a18-20.
52. Gotthard Strohmaier, 'Dura mater, Pia mater. Die Geschichte zweier anatomischer Termini', *Med. hist. J.*, V (1970) 201-16.
53. For this problem see Theodor Puschmann, *Alexander von Tralles*, Bd. I, Vienna 1878, 148-56.
54. Browne, *Medicine*, 113.
55. Paulus Aegin. III, 6, I (vol. I, 144 ff. Heiberg).
56. David Neil MacKenzie, *A Concise Pahlavi Dictionary*, London 1971, 74; 87.
57. cf. *Ḥamāsa* of Abū-Tammām, 819 v. 3 (ed. Freytag); Jirān al-ʿAwd, XII, 20 (p. 38, I); Ruʾba, LIV, 173 (ed. Ahlwardt).
58. Jābir ibn-Ḥayyān, *Kitāb as-Sumūm*, ed. Alfred Siggel, Wiesbaden 1958, fol. 101a6; Ikhwān aṣ-Ṣafā', Beirut 1957, II, 319, 6.
59. Abū-Manṣūr al-Jawālīqī, *Kitāb al-Muʿarrab min al-kalām al-aʿjamī*, ed. Aḥmad Muḥammad Shākir, Cairo 1942, 45.
60. Muḥammad ibn-al-Ḥasan ibn-Durayd al-Azdī, *Kitāb Jamharat al-lugha*, III, Hyderabad 1345, 386a10f.
61. Galen, 'On the Parts of Medicine, On Cohesive Causes . . .', ed. Malcolm Lyons (*CMG*, Suppl. Or., II), Berlin 1969, 70, 10; Rāzī, *Ḥāwī*, I, 202; 219; XV, 67; Ibn-Sīnā, *Qānūn*, I, 302 ff.
62. Translation by Ludwig Edelstein.

63. *De locis affectis*, III, 10 (vol. VIII, 190 Kühn).
64. Orib., *Coll. med. Libr. inc.* 29, 9.
65. *Kitāb Siyāsat aṣ-ṣibyān*, ed. Muḥammad al-Ḥabīb al-Hīla, Tunis 1968, 61, 3.
66. Manfred Ullmann, in: *Med. hist. J.*, IX (1974) 30-7.
67. Charles Homer Haskins, *Studies in the History of Mediaeval Science* (Harvard Historical Studies vol. XXVII), Cambridge, Mass. 1924, 206-9.
68. *Galen On Anatomical Procedures, the later books*, a translation by the late W. L. H. Duckworth, ed. M. C. Lyons and B. Towers, Cambridge 1962.
69. 'Galen Über die Verschiedenheit der homoiomeren Körperteile, in arabischer Übersetzung zum erstenmal herausgegeben, übersetzt und erläutert' von Gotthard Strohmaier (*CMG*, Supplementum Orientale III) Berlin 1970.
70. *Galen On Medical Experience*, first edition of the Arabic version with English translation and notes by Richard Walzer, London – New York – Toronto 1944; rep. 1946 and 1947.
71. Karl Deichgräber, *Die griechische Empirikerschule. Sammlung der Fragmente und Darstellung der Lehre*, Berlin 1930; Ludwig Edelstein, 'Empiricism and Scepticism in the Teaching of the Greek Empiricist School', in: Edelstein, *Ancient Medicine*, 195-203.
72. Galen, *De locis affectis*, V, 8 (vol. VIII, 354f. Kühn).
73. Galen, *De locis affectis*, III, 6 (vol. VIII, 160ff. Kühn).
74. Rāzī, *Ḥāwī*, I, 94f.
75. Manfred Ullmann, 'Die Krankengeschichten des Rufus von Ephesos', *Akten des VII. Kongresses für Arabistik und Islamwissenschaft* (Göttingen 1974), Abhandl. d. Akad. d. Wiss. in Göttingen, phil.-hist. Klasse, Dritte Folge, Nr. 98, 1976, 364-71.
76. Flashar, *Melancholie*, 84-104.
77. Galen, *De locis affectis*, III, 10 (vol. VIII, 179-93 Kühn).
78. Manfred Ullmann, 'Die Schrift des Rufus "De infantium curatione" und das Problem der Autorenlemmata in den "Collectiones medicae" des Oreibasios', *Med. hist. J.*, X (1975) 165-90.
79. Manfred Ullmann, 'Neues zu den diätetischen Schriften des Rufus von Ephesos', *Med. hist. J.*, IX (1974) 23-40.

Chapter Three

1. *The Book of the Ten Treatises on the Eye Ascribed to Hunain ibn Is-hâq. The earliest existing systematic textbook of Ophthalmology.* The Arabic text edited from the only two known manuscripts, with an English translation and glossary by Max Meyerhof, Cairo 1928.

2. Giuseppe Celentano, 'Il trattatello di Ḥunain Ibn Isḥāq sulla profilassi e terapia dei denti', *Annali dell'Istituto Orientale di Napoli*, XXXV (1975) 45-80; Rainer Degen, 'Eine weitere Handschrift von Ḥunain ibn Isḥāqs Schrift über die Zahnheilkunde', ibid., XXXVI (1976) 236-43.
3. Rainer Degen, 'A Further Note on some Syriac Manuscripts in the Mingana Collection', *Journal of Semitic Studies*, XVII (1972) 213-17.
4. Paul Sbath, 'Le Livre des caractères de Qosṭâ ibn Loûqâ', *Bulletin de l'Institut d'Égypte*, XXIII (1941) 103-69.
5. Max Meyerhof, 'Thirty-three Clinical Observations by Rhazes (circa 900 A.D.)', *Isis*, XXIII (1935) 321-72.
6. *Kitāb al-Ḥāwī fi ṭ-ṭibb* (Continens of Rhazes), Part I-XXIII, Hyderabad – Deccan, 1955–71.
7. Lenn Evan Goodman, 'The Epicurean Ethic of Muḥammad ibn Zakariyâ' ar-Râzî', *Studia Islamica*, XXXIV (1971) 5-26.
8. Cyril Elgood, *EI*², I, 381 a.
9. Translation by Martin S. Spink and Geoffrey L. Lewis, *Albucasis On Surgery and Instruments*. A definitive edition of the Arabic text with English translation and commentary, Berkeley and Los Angeles 1973, 2.
10. William E. Gohlman, *The Life of Ibn Sina. A Critical Edition and Annotated Translation* (Studies in Islamic Philosophy and Science) Albany, New York 1974 (cf. *Der Islam*, LII [1975] 148-51).
11. Francesca Lucchetta, *Il medico e filosofo Bellunese Andrea Alpago* (†1522), *traduttore di Avicenna. Profilo biografico*, Padua 1964.
12. Roger Arnaldez, *EI*², III, 909-20.
13. Friedrich W. Zimmermann, *Der Islam*, LI (1974) 165 f.
14. Georges Vajda, *EI*², III, 876-8; Fred Rosner, 'Maimonides the physician: a bibliography', *Bull. Hist. Med.*, XLIII (1969) 221-235.
15. *The Medical Aphorisms of Moses Maimonides*, translated and edited by Fred Rosner and Suessman Muntner (Studies in Judaica vol. III), vol. I. II, New York 1970.71, second printing 1973.
16. *Moses Maimonides' Two Treatises on the Regimen of Health*, translated from the Arabic and edited in accordance with the Hebrew and Latin versions by Ariel Bar-Sela, H. E. Hoff a.o. (Transactions of the American Philosophical Society N.S. LIV, 4), Philadelphia 1964; Felix Klein-Franke, 'Der hippokratische und der maimonidische Arzt', *Freiburger Zeitschrift für Philosophie und Theologie*, XVII (1970) 442-9.

17. Claude Cahen, '‘Abdallaṭīf al-Baghdādī—portraitiste et historien de son temps. Extraits inédits de ses Mémoires', *Bulletin d'Études Orientales*, XXIII (1970) 101-28.
18. Max Meyerhof and Joseph Schacht, *The Theologus Autodidactus of Ibn al-Nafīs*, Oxford 1968; Josef van Ess, *Orientalische Literaturzeitung*, LXVIII (1973) 487-9.
19. *The Natural History of Aleppo. Containing a Description of the City, and the Principal Natural Productions in its Neighbourhood: Together with an Account of the Climate, Inhabitants and Diseases; Particularly of the Plague.* By Alexander Russell, M.D. The Second Edition, revised, enlarged, and illustrated with Notes. By Pat. Russell, M.D., vol. I. II, London 1794.
20. Robert Ricard, 'Médecine et médecins à Arzila (1508–1539)', *Hespéris*, XXVI (1939) 171-8.
21. C.E. Daniëls, 'La Version orientale, arabe et turque, des deux premiers livres de Herman Boerhaave. Étude bibliographique', *Janus*, XVII (1912) 295-312.
22. Ernst Julius Gurlt, in: *Biographisches Lexikon der hervorragenden Ärzte*, vol. II, 1930, 55f.
23. Karl Hummel, 'Die Entwicklung der neuzeitlichen Naturwissenschaft in Iran', *Die Welt des Orients*, VI (1971) 240-54.
24. J.B. Piot Bey, 'La mission Pasteur de 1883 pour l'étude du choléra en Égypte', *Bulletin de l'Institut d'Égypte*, V (1923) 1-7.
25. Henry E. Sigerist, *A History of Medicine*, vol. I: *Primitive and Archaic Medicine*, New York 1951, 25; M. Zubair Siddiqi, 'The Unani Tibb (Greek Medicine) in India', *Islamic Culture*, XLII (1968) 161-72; Hakim Mohammed Said, 'Traditional Greco-Arabic and Modern Western Medicine: Conflict or Symbiosis', in: *Islam und Abendland. Geschichte und Gegenwart* (Universität Bern, Kulturhistorische Vorlesungen 1974/75, ed. André Mercier), Berne and Frankfurt 1976, 221-61; *Asian Medical Systems: A Comparative Study*, ed. Charles Leslie, Berkeley–Los Angeles–London 1976.
26. Moritz Steinschneider, *Die europäischen Übersetzungen aus dem Arabischen bis Mitte des 17. Jahrhunderts* (Sitzungsberichte der Kaiserlichen Akademie der Wissenschaften in Wien, phil.-hist. Klasse), 1904. 05, rep. Graz 1956; Charles Homer Haskins, *Studies in the History of Mediaeval Science* (Harvard Historical Studies vol. XXVII) Cambridge, Mass. 1924; Heinrich Schipperges, 'Die frühen Übersetzer der arabischen Medizin in chronologischer Sicht', *Sudhoffs Archiv*, XXXIX (1955) 53-93; id., *Die Assimilation der arabischen Medizin durch das lateinische Mittelalter* (Sudhoffs Archiv, Beihefte, Heft 3), Wiesbaden 1964; B. Ben Yahia, *EI*^{2}, II, 59f. (s.v. Constantinus Africanus).

27. Heinrich Schipperges, *Ideologie und Historiographie des Arabismus* (Sudhoffs Archiv, Beihefte, Heft 1), Wiesbaden 1961.

Chapter Four

1. Majūsī, *Malakī*, I, 9.
2. ibid., 15 ff.
3. ibid., 18 ff.
4. ibid., 43 ff.
5. For the different sorts of the yellow bile cf. Siegel, *Galen's Physiology*, 220.
6. Galen, *De naturalibus facultatibus*, II, 9 (vol. II, 125 ff. Kühn).
7. Majūsī, *Malakī*, I, 47.
8. The concept of the natural faculties found in Majūsī, *Malakī*, I, 130 ff., corresponds to Galen, *De temperamentis*, III, 1 (p. 90 f. Helmreich), but in Galen's works also a different concept is to be met with, see Temkin, *Galenism*, 89.
9. Temkin, *Galenism*, 89.
10. Majūsī, *Malakī*, I, 138 ff.
11. ibid., 143 ff.
12. Hermann Siebeck, *Geschichte der Psychologie*, Theil 1, 2. Abtheilung, Gotha 1884, 130-60; Fridolf Kudlien, 'Pneumatische Ärzte', in: *RE*, Suppl., XI (1968) col. 1097-1108.
13. Owsei Temkin, 'On Galen's Pneumatology', *Gesnerus*, VIII (1951) 180-9; cf. also the chapter 'The Two Types of Pneuma', in: Siegel, *Galen's Physiology*, 183 ff.
14. Walther Sudhoff, 'Die Lehre von den Hirnventrikeln in textlicher und graphischer Tradition des Altertums und Mittelalters', *Sudhoffs Archiv*, VII (1913) 149-205.
15. Majūsī, *Malakī*, I, 114 ff.
16. ibid., 68 ff.
17. ibid., 107 ff.
18. I likewise shall not dwell upon the question whether Galen had already expounded the idea of a transference of blood through the pulmonary artery and vein, a view which is held by Rudolph E. Siegel in his book on *Galen's System of Physiology*, 30 ff. The important thing is only the knowledge possessed by al-Majūsī and the other Arab physicians of their time.
19. Max Meyerhof and Joseph Schacht, *The Theologus Autodidactus of Ibn al-Nafīs*, Oxford 1968.
20. Max Meyerhof, 'Ibn an-Nafīs und seine Theorie des Lungenkreislaufs', *Quellen und Studien zur Geschichte der Naturwissenschaften und der Medizin*, IV (1935) 37-88. For further literature see Ullmann, *Medizin*, 173-6; Siegel, *Galen's Physiology*, 65 f.

21. Albert Zakī Iskandar, *A Catalogue of Arabic Manuscripts on Medicine and Science in the Wellcome Historical Medical Library*, London 1967, 181-3.
22. Owsei Temkin, 'Was Servetus influenced by Ibn an-Nafīs?', *Bull. Hist. Med.*, VIII (1940) 731-4; Joseph Schacht, 'Ibn al-Nafīs, Servetus and Colombo', *Al-Andalus*, XXII (1957) 317-336.
23. vol. IX, 168 Littré.
24. Majūsī, *Malakī*, I, 110.
25. ibid., 114, 4ff.
26. Walter Artelt, 'Ossa mandibulae inferioris duo', *Sudhoffs Archiv*, XXXIX (1955) 193-215.

Chapter Five

1. MS. Munich 805, fol. 89b-120b. Isḥāq ibn ʿImrān, *Maqāla fī l-Mālīḫūliyā* (*Abhandlung über die Melancholie*) *und Constantini Africani Libri duo de melancholia.* Vergleichende kritische arabisch-lateinische Parallelausgabe. Deutsche Übersetzung des Arabischen Textes . . . von Karl Garbers, Hamburg 1977.

1a. cf. Parviz Morewedge, *The* Metaphysica *of Avicenna*, London 1973, 172 (Editor's note).

2. Owsei Temkin, *The Falling Sickness : a History of Epilepsy from the Greeks to the Beginnings of Modern Neurology*, 2nd ed., Baltimore and London 1971. Index s.v. Melancholy.
3. Flashar, *Melancholie*, 76f.
4. Galen, *De locis affectis*, III, 10 (vol. VIII, 179-93 Kühn).
5. Majūsī, *Malakī*, I, 332ff.
6. Flashar, *Melancholie*, 129f.
7. Majūsī, *Malakī*, I, 379f.
8. Galen, *De locis affectis*, VI, 3 (vol. VIII, 394ff. Kühn).
9. Hans-Jürgen Thies, *Der Diabetestraktat ʿAbd al-Laṭīf al-Baġdādī's. Untersuchungen zur Geschichte des Krankheitsbildes in der arabischen Medizin* (Bonner Orientalistische Studien, N.S. XXI) Bonn 1971.
10. Samuel Miklos Stern, in: *Islamic Studies*, I, 1 (1962) 61.
11. Rāzī, *Ḥāwī*, XIX, 150.
12. ibid., 130.
13. Friedrich Fülleborn, in: *Handbuch der pathogenen Mikroorganismen*, 3. Auflage, hsgb. von W. Kolle, R. Kraus, P. Uhlenhut, VI. Band, II. Teil, Jena–Berlin–Vienna 1929, 1196-1223.
14. Galen, *De locis affectis*, VI, 3 (vol. VIII, 393 Kühn).
15. Paulus Aegin., IV, 58 (vol. I, 387f. Heiberg).
16. Rāzī, *Ḥāwī*, XI, 290.

17. Vol. XIX, 449 Kühn.
18. Vol. XIV, 790f. Kühn.
19. Majūsī, *Malakī*, I, 314; II, 209.
20. Ed. Spink and Lewis, p. 600f.
21. Ullmann, *Medizin*, 124.
22. Rāzī, *Ḥāwī*, XI, 292.
23. ibid., 294.
24. ibid., 292.
25. ibid., 293.
26. ibid.
27. Ibn-Sīnā, *Qānūn*, II, 76.
28. Karl Meier, 'Über den Medina-Wurm', *Sudhoffs Archiv*, XXX (1937–8) 69-77.
29. Majūsī, *Malakī*, I, 309f.
30. Paul Richter, 'Beiträge zur Geschichte der Pocken bei den Arabern', *Sudhoffs Archiv*, V (1912) 311-31.
31. Georg Sticker, *Das Heufieber und verwandte Störungen. Klinik der Idiopathien*, 2. Aufl., Vienna and Leipzig 1912, 14-17.
32. Friedrun R. Hau, 'Razis Gutachten über Rosenschnupfen', *Med. hist. J.*, X (1975) 94-102.

Chapter Six

1. Galen, *De differentiis febrium*, I, 3 (vol. VII, 279 Kühn).
2. Ibn-al-Kalbī, in: *K. al-Aghānī*, IX, 178/XI, 43.
3. Al-Bukhārī, *Ṣaḥīḥ*, Ṭibb nr. LIII, 19 and 30.
4. G. H. A. Juynboll, *The Authenticity of the Tradition Literature: Discussions in Modern Egypt*, Leiden 1969, 140f.
5. Wensinck, *Concordance*, III, 327; IV, 158f.
6. Ibrāhīm an-Naẓẓām, cf. Josef van Ess, 'Ein unbekanntes Fragment des Naẓẓām', *Der Orient in der Forschung. Festschrift für Otto Spies*, Wiesbaden 1967, 172; 180f.
7. Majūsī, *Malakī*, I, 310f.
8. ibid., II, 64 paen. ff.
9. Qazwīnī, *'Ajā'ib al-makhlūqāt*, 364, 20ff.
10. Jāḥiẓ, *Ḥayawān*, IV, 73/220.
11. Majūsī, *Malakī*, I, 168ff.; II, 62ff.
12. This complex of symptoms was described first by Rufus, see Paulus Aegin., II, 35, 1 (vol. I, 108 Heiberg).
13. Al-Majūsī's source here is the Thucydides quotation by Galen, *De differentiis febrium*, I, 6 (vol. VII, 290 Kühn).
14. I, 6 (vol. VII, 290 Kühn).
15. Majūsī, *Malakī*, II, 62-5.
16. Galen, *De simpl. med. temp. ac fac.*, IX, 1, 4 (vol. XII, 191 Kühn).

17. Haeser, *Lehrbuch*, III, 16-18.
18. Ibn-al-Ukhuwwa, *Maʿālim*, ch. XLII.
19. Michael Walter Dols, *The Black Death in the Middle East*, Diss. Princeton 1971.
20. Erwin H. Ackerknecht, *Rudolf Virchow, Doctor, Statesman, Anthropologist*, Madison 1953, 106ff.
21. Michael Dols, 'Ibn al-Wardī's Risālah al-naba' ʿan al-waba', a Translation of a Major Source for the History of the Black Death in the Middle East', in: *Near Eastern Numismatics, Iconography, Epigraphy and History. Studies in Honor of George C. Miles*, Beirut 1974, 443-55.
22. Rachel Arié, 'Un Opuscule grenadin sur la peste noire de 1348: La "Naṣīḥa" de Muḥammad al-Šaqūrī', *Boletín de la Asociación Española de Orientalistas*, III (1967) 189-99.
23. ʿAlī ibn-Sahl aṭ-Ṭabarī, *Firdaws al-ḥikma*, 428.
24. J. Bosch-Vilá, EI^2, III, 835ff.
25. *El libro del ʿAmal man ṭabba li-man ḥabba de Muḥammad b. ʿAbdallāh bi al-Jaṭīb*, texto árabe, con glosario, editado por Maria Concepción Vázquez de Benito, Salamanca 1972.
26. Marcus Joseph Müller, 'Ibnulkhatîbs Bericht über die Pest', *Sitzungsberichte der königl. bayer. Akademie der Wissenschaften zu München*, 1863, vol. II, 1-34.
27. Gustave Edmund von Grunebaum, *Medieval Islam: a Study in Cultural Orientation*, 2nd ed., Chicago 1953, 335f.
28. Diepgen, *Medizin*, I, 262.
29. Jacqueline Sublet, 'La Peste prise aux rets de la jurisprudence. Le traité d'Ibn Ḥağar al-ʿAsqalānī sur la peste', *Studia Islamica*, XXXIII (1971) 141-9.
30. Robert Ricard, *Hespéris* (1939) 177f.

Chapter Seven

1. Majūsī, *Malakī*, I, 14.
2. ibid., 152-217.
3. Peter H. Niebyl, 'The Non-Naturals', *Bull. Hist. Med.*, XLV (1971) 486-92.
4. Ludwig Edelstein, 'The Dietetics of Antiquity', in: Edelstein, *Ancient Medicine*, 303-16.
5. Hippocrates, *Epidemics*, VI, 8. 7-10 (vol. V, 344ff. Littré).
6. Georg Harig, *Bestimmung der Intensität im medizinischen System Galens*, Berlin 1974, 89f.
7. Majūsī, *Malakī*, I, 179ff.
8. Albertus von Haller, *Bibliotheca botanica*, vol. I, Tiguri, 1771, 182.

9. Majūsī, *Malakī*, II, 84-152.
10. See Georg Harig (n.6).

Chapter Eight

1. Ludwig Edelstein, 'Greek Medicine in its Relation to Religion and Magic', *Bull. Hist. Med.*, V (1937) 201-46, reprinted in: Edelstein, *Ancient Medicine*, 205-46.
2. Paul Diepgen, 'Volksmedizin und wissenschaftliche Heilkunde', in: *Volk und Volkstum*, II (1937) 45, reprinted in: Grabner, *Volksmedizin*, 210f.
3. Heinrich Vorwahl, in: Grabner, *Volksmedizin*, 261.
4. Rāzī, *Ḥāwī*, X, 102.
5. ibid., XII, 225.
6. ibid., XIX, 254.
7. Ms. Gotha, 1975, fol. 41aff. (Maqāla I, ch. 51).
8. Quoted by at-Tamīmī, *Kitāb al-Murshid*, in: Ibn-al-Bayṭār, *Kitāb al-Jāmiʿ*, III, 10.
9. Hovorka-Kronfeld, I, 14-18 (s.v. Alraun); 286-8 (s.v. Mandragora); Heinrich Vorwahl, 'Deutsche Volksmedizin in Vergangenheit und Gegenwart', in: *Studien zur religiösen Volkskunde*, Abt. B, H. 9, Dresden–Leipzig 1939, 27, reprinted in: Grabner, *Volksmedizin*, 251f.
10. Jutta Schönfeld, *Über die Steine* (Islamkundliche Untersuchungen, Bd. XXXVIII), Freiburg 1976, 80 and 171.
11. Ullmann, *Medizin*, 311-13.
12. Manfred Ullmann, 'Die arabische Überlieferung der Kyranis des Hermes Trismegistos', *Proceedings of the VIth Congress of Arabic and Islamic Studies* (Visby–Stockholm 1972), Stockholm–Leiden 1975, 196-200.
13. Felix Klein-Franke, 'Die Ursachen der Krisen bei akuten Krankheiten. Eine wiederentdeckte Schrift al-Kindī's', *Israel Oriental Studies*, V (1975) 161-88.
14. Rāzī, *Ḥāwī*, XVIII, 39f.
15. Oskar Rescher, 'Studien über den Inhalt von 1001 Nacht', *Der Islam*, IX (1919) 36.
16. Samira Kortantamer, *Ägypten und Syrien zwischen 1317 und 1341 in der Chronik des Mufaḍḍal b. Abī l-Faḍā'il*, Freiburg 1973, 256f.
17. Charles Pellat, *EI*², I, 628.
18. ʿArīb ibn Saʿīd al-Kātib al-Qurṭubi, *Le Livre de la génération du foetus et le traitement des femmes enceintes et des nouveau-nés*, publié, traduit et annoté par Henri Jahier et Noureddine Abdelkader, Algiers 1956, 38f.

19. Majūsī, *Malakī*, 1, 120f.
20. ʿArīb (see n. 18), 85-7.
21. Ibn-al-Khaṭīb, *Muqniʿa*, 2, 10ff.
22. August Ferdinand Mehren, 'Vues d'Avicenne sur l'astrologie', *Muséon*, III (1884) 383-403.

INDEX

The Arabic article al-, *with its variants*, an-, ash-, *etc.*, *is neglected in the alphabetical arrangement*

Rufus of Ephesus, 13, 21-3, 31, 34-40, 42-3, 76, 80, 91
Russell, Alexander, 49

Ṣakhr al-Ghayy, 4
Saladin, 47, 99
Salicetti, Guilielmo, 45
Ṣāliḥ ibn-Naṣr-Allāh, *see* Ibn-Sallūm
Salmawayh ibn-Bunān, 34
Salomon ben-Nathan Hameati, 34
as-Samarqandī, Najīb-ad-Dīn, 25, 99
Sergius of Rēsh-ʿAynā, 16
Servetus, Michael, 69
Shams-ad-Dawla Abū-Ṭāhir, 45
Shānāq, 20
Shāpūr I, son of Ardashīr, 16-17
ash-Shaqūrī, Muḥammad, 92
Shemʿōn d-Ṭaybūtheh, 16
Shlēmōn, 16
Simon, Max, 32
Soranus of Ephesus, 15, 21, 82
Stephanus (philosopher), 8
Stephanus (physician), 13
Stephen of Pisa, 54
Ṣubḥī-Zāde ʿAbd-al-ʿAzīz, 51
as-Sukkarī, 29
Suśruta, 20, 41

aṭ-Ṭabarī, Aḥmad ibn-Muḥammad, 14
aṭ-Ṭabarī, ʿAlī ibn-Sahl, 20, 22, 41, 83, 108, 111-12
at-Takrītī, Yaḥyā ibn-Jarīr, 111
at-Tamīmī, Muḥammad ibn-Aḥmad, 48, 110
Teucrus, 17
Thābit ibn-Qurra, 9, 11, 78, 88, 95
Themison of Laodicaea, 21
Theophrastus, 78
Thucydides, 86
Tiyādhūq, 6

ʿUmar ibn-ʿAbd-al-ʿAzīz, 8
ʿUrwa ibn-az-Zubayr, 5

Vāgbhata, 20, 41
Valerian (emperor), 17
de Valverde, Giovanni, 69
Vesalius, Andreas, 22, 43
Vettius Valens, 17
Virchow, Rudolf, 91

Wahb ibn-Munabbih, 5
al-Walīd ibn-ʿAbd-al-Malik, 5
Walzer, Richard, 33
al-Wāthiq, 41
Wyman, Morill, 84

Xenocrates of Aphrodisias, 19, 42, 108
Xenocrates of Ephesus, 14
Xenophon, 38

Yaḥyā ibn-al-Biṭrīq, 9
Yaḥyā ibn-Khālid al-Barmakī, 20
al-Yaʿqūbī, 11
Yōḥannān bar Serāphyōn, 16
Yūḥannā, *see* Ibn-Māsawayh
Yūnus ibn-Ḥabīb, 6

az-Zahrāwī, 14, 24, 26, 44-5, 52, 54, 82
Zayn-al-ʿArab al-Miṣrī, 69
Ziyādat-Allāh 111, 72

(b) *Subject-matter*